THE WHOLE-BODY GUIDE TO GUT HEALTH

the WHOLE-BODY **Guide** to Gut Health

HEAL YOUR GUT THROUGH
DIET, EXERCISE, AND STRESS REDUCTION

Heidi Moretti, MS, RD

Illustrations by
Donna Grethen

ROCKRIDGE
PRESS

For general information on our other products and services or to obtain technical
support, please contact our Customer Care Department within the United States at
(866) 744-2665, or outside the United States at (510) 253-0500.

Interior and Cover Designer: Heather Krakora
Art Producer: Meg Baggott
Editor: Justin Hartung
Production Editor: Andrew Yackira

Illustrations © 2021 Donna Grethen

Author photo courtesy of AthenaPhotography.com

ISBN: Print 978-1-64876-616-9 | eBook 978-1-64876-115-7

R0

To my parents,
Don and Janet DeBoo,
who always encourage me to
fully experience everything
around me, especially nature,
and to examine the status quo.

Contents

Introduction

Welcome! By reading this book, you are taking your first step toward healing your gut. When your gut feels good, it is so much more than just a "gut feeling"; this is because your gut health is closely connected to all systems in your body, and what you eat has a huge impact on your overall health.

In my many years of clinical experience, I've found that improving gut health is the single best way to help my clients feel better. After all, gut issues are often the root cause of many ailments and diseases. By focusing on the gut in a holistic way, my clients often start to notice that their depression symptoms lift or their aches and pains go away. Perhaps their long-standing heartburn disappears or their energy gets a boost. This is because improving your gut health by eating good food, taking key supplements (when needed), and attending to your physical and emotional well-being provides your body with the best opportunity to heal.

On a personal level, I've benefited tremendously by focusing on my gut. From improvements in skin conditions like eczema to boosts in my mood, energy, and memory, gut health has made all the difference in how I look and feel.

I am so excited to help you with your gut health, too. The steps that I discuss in the book are the optimum way to get your gut—and your whole body—on the road to recovery. The best part is that when you embark on this journey, you will feel better, which will cause a positive snowball effect on your whole outlook. Even if things don't go perfectly right away, I provide you with ways to troubleshoot your symptoms, so you can stay the course and achieve better health.

I break down the basics of gut health for you in this book, from identifying parts of the digestive tract and explaining their functions to how nutrients and healthy bacteria can support healing. I also explain the gut's relationship with every part of your body and mind and how, by recognizing this, you can enhance your health holistically.

Many digestive diseases are related to the food you eat. I explain how these conditions can be improved by making some simple changes in your diet, as well as when to seek help from your doctor. I provide lists of foods that support gut health, foods that you should eat in smaller amounts, and foods that commonly cause digestive issues and should be avoided. By following this guide, you can expect to alleviate most, if not all, of the digestive distress that is caused by the pitfalls of modern diets.

I also provide you with easy, practical exercises, including yoga and meditation, that you can do almost anywhere without expensive gym memberships. You will also learn about how to easily incorporate lifestyle strategies that are fun and improve gut health.

Last but not least, the most awesome part of this book are the 50 tasty recipes that are easy to make and help nourish the gut. I've also included a two-week meal plan for getting started on your holistic gut health journey.

These recipes and tips are the template for your healing journey and for the rest of your life. You won't want to go back to your old ways of eating once you experience how much better you can feel!

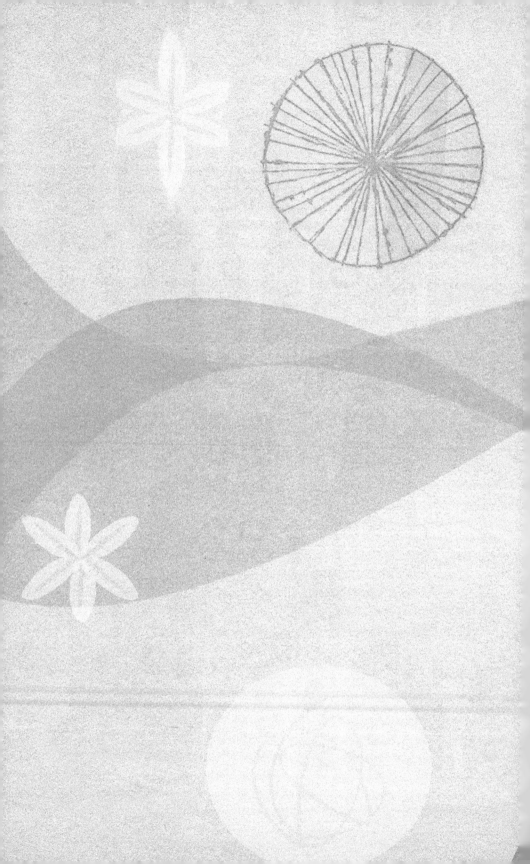

Part One

Get to Know Your Gut

CHAPTER 1

Your Gut, Explained

Your "gut" is composed of your digestive organs and the microbes that live within them. It is responsible for many crucial functions in your body. Not only does it manage the processes involved in the digestion and absorption of nutrients, but it also protects you from harmful "outside invaders." An astounding 70 percent of your immune cells live in your gut. This means that a large part of your response to bacteria, viruses, and allergens is controlled by your digestive tract. Additionally, your gut interacts with other organs and systems within your body, including the nervous system, brain, and heart.

In this chapter, I'll demystify the gut by identifying its various parts, explaining how they work, and clarifying how the gut connects to and works with different parts of the body.

Gut Basics

You may be surprised to learn that when you see or smell food, the "mouthwatering" sensation you feel is the beginning of the digestive process. The secretion of saliva that begins with sensory stimulation then increases when you begin chewing your food. Saliva contains enzymes that help break down what you eat. From there, a variety of organs from the esophagus to the liver support digestion, but the major players are the stomach, intestines, and enteric nervous system. A basic understanding of how these three components work is crucial to improving and maintaining your gut health.

STOMACH

Located between your esophagus and small intestine, your stomach makes enzymes to help break down food. It also produces hydrochloric acid, which helps you absorb important vitamins and minerals and is critical for digesting proteins. Too much hydrochloric acid can reflux, or flow backward, into the esophagus, causing a feeling of heartburn. Too little acid can also cause heartburn and indigestion. This is because low acid, or acid deficiency, causes your foods to be inadequately digested, which can throw your whole system out of balance. Acid deficiency can cause other issues as well, including gas, bloating, belching, fatigue, digestive system infections, and nutrient deficiencies.

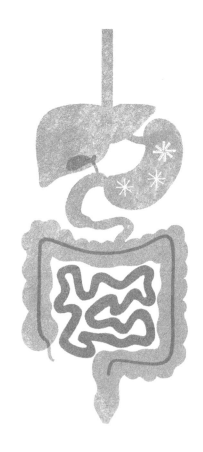

INTESTINES

Your intestines act like an orchestra conductor, sending signals about digestion to your whole body. When food leaves your stomach, acid-neutralizing particles, bile, and enzymes are released from your gallbladder and pancreas. These help protect your intestines from acid and advance the digestive activity that occurs there. After digestion, the main job of the small intestines is to facilitate the absorption of nutrients from your food into the bloodstream.

The lining of your intestines, or epithelium, acts as a gatekeeper during this process. It discerns whether a digested particle should be allowed into the body or not. When healthy, the epithelium makes antimicrobial substances and has a thick mucus layer above it, which helps slough off harmful germs and toxins. It also contains lymphocytes, which communicate with the immune system and help decide whether a digested substance is a friend or foe.

Your large intestine is responsible for absorbing water and electrolytes, managing food waste, and reabsorbing substances like bile. Basically, the large intestine helps do the cleanup work and ensures that your fluids are balanced. Home to trillions of bacteria, the large intestine also plays a big role in how your immune system functions, because these bacteria act like a communication highway, passing information from your gut to your immune system and your brain.

ENTERIC NERVOUS SYSTEM

The portion of your nervous system located in the digestive tract is called the enteric nervous system. It reaches from the esophagus to the bowels and connects everything in between, including the stomach, the pancreas, and even the small arteries that directly receive nutrients from the intestines.

Have you ever had a "gut" feeling about a decision or felt butterflies in your stomach? That's because your enteric nervous system connects to your central processing center—your brain. The enteric nervous system is sometimes even referred to as "the second brain." If you feel an emotion—good, bad, or otherwise—it often affects your gut. It works the other way, too: If your gut isn't healthy, it can cause mood problems and brain fog.

Finally, the enteric nervous system controls the muscle movements of your intestines, which make it possible for your body to remove waste. The healthier your overall system, the more efficiently those muscles operate.

Meet Your Microbiome

The unique assortment of organisms that coexist within your body are collectively called your microbiome. Consisting of bacteria, viruses, and fungi, your gut's microbiome contains around 100 trillion cells—10 times more than the rest of your body. These tiny copilots in your gut, called microbiota or gut flora, control a lot of what happens in your body, including your digestion, nerves, brain, muscles, and more.

Your gut flora helps digest food by breaking it down into smaller particles, but it does much more than that: Healthy bacteria in the gut can help fight and kill harmful microbes and synthesize some vitamins, such as B vitamins and vitamin K. By breaking down some kinds of fibers, good bacteria also provide fuel to your intestinal cells, which helps protect your epithelial lining. According to the research journal *Frontiers in Immunology*, this protection of the epithelial lining may reduce your chances of allergic reactions and inflammatory diseases and can help you develop immune tolerances. Furthermore, your gut flora regulates the frequency of your bowel movements, improves stool consistency, reduces diarrhea, and can even help prevent irritable bowel syndrome by fending off bad bacteria and helping your body absorb nutrients and electrolytes from your diet.

From the second you are born, your microbiome is exposed to a wide variety of bacteria and microbes, or "bugs," from your diet and your environment. Medications such as antibiotics, stomach acid drugs, and diabetes medication, as well as exposure to toxins including pesticides, artificial sweeteners, and heavy metals like mercury, can damage your microbiome. However, the type and diversity of food you eat also affects your microbiome and can even change how you feel. That's good news, because it means you can make a few easy adjustments and experience a meaningful improvement in your health.

One way to increase the diversity of your microbiome and improve your overall health is to add fermented foods to your diet. Many fermented foods, such as yogurt, sauerkraut, kombucha, and aged cheese, are rich in probiotics, or beneficial bacteria. And probiotics benefit your overall health in big ways. A review of five research papers published in the journal *Nutrients* concluded that probiotic consumption is associated with significant reduction in depression symptoms. Consumption of probiotics is even emerging as a safe approach to reduce the severity of nonalcoholic fatty liver disease. Studies in the *World Journal of Gastroenterology* and *Journal of Neuroinflammation* suggest that probiotics may even reduce the severity of the debilitating effects of multiple sclerosis.

Everything Is Connected

Thinking about the health of every individual system in your body can be overwhelming. Instead, it can be easier—and even more effective—to focus on the big picture. This is because of one simple fact: In your body, everything is connected. This is the fundamental concept of holistic health, and it means that you treat the whole person rather than a single part. When you make one positive change, it can create a beneficial ripple effect throughout your whole body. This is especially true of your gut, which can affect your nervous system, your heart, your liver, your brain, your hormones, and even your skin.

NERVOUS SYSTEM

You've already learned about the way in which your gut and nervous system interact. In fact, according to the latest research, neurological autoimmune diseases like multiple sclerosis have links to altered gut bacteria. In the guts of patients with multiple sclerosis and other neurological conditions, you'll usually find an increase in harmful bacteria. This can create a cascade of damaging inflammation in your nervous system and in the whole body, which perceives this bacterial imbalance as a threat.

HEART

Much like your nervous system, your heart and blood vessels are constantly receiving information from your belly. In fact, the effects of the gut on your heart can be almost immediate because of the remarkably close connection between your blood supply and your digestive tract. The nutrients absorbed from the food passing through your intestines, as well as signals from your microbiome, instantly make an impression on your heart and blood vessels. The immune system then examines the contents and decides whether to sound the alarm to your heart or accept the food as nourishment.

LIVER

The liver has many functions, but its main job within the digestive system is to process the nutrients absorbed from the small intestine. Bile is secreted from the liver into the small intestine, where it plays an important role in digesting fat and some vitamins. Your liver is responsible for detoxifying your body and packaging and distributing nutrients to other organs. In this way, your liver connects to the health of your whole body, including the gut.

BRAIN

Brain health is closely tied to the health of your gut. For example, when you make a positive change in your diet, you may be able to think more clearly, and your mood may improve. Most "happy brain" substances like serotonin are primarily made in the gut. Your sleep quality can be directly influenced by your food and gut health, too. According to the journal *PLoS One,* next time you consider sleep medication, you may want to address gut health first to see if it is at the root of your sleep problems.

HORMONES

Hormones are complex but can be improved by many of the same diet and lifestyle changes that help your gut, brain, liver, and heart. Your immune system, which is located primarily in your gut, strongly influences hormones such as thyroid hormones, insulin, estrogen, and testosterone. For example, food intolerances cause inflammation in the gut, which may then impair the function of the thyroid or even affect insulin production. On the positive side, when you eat certain foods, like broccoli, they may help reduce harmful forms of estrogen and promote healthy testosterone levels.

SKIN

Perhaps the most surprising of all connections is between gut health and the skin. Some health experts, like Dr. Cassandra Quave from Emory University and *International Journal of Colorectal Disease*, have described the skin as a "window to your gut health." On a personal note, by identifying my own food intolerances and gut imbalances and correcting them, I improved my skin tone, acne, and eczema. Food changes made a bigger difference for my skin and overall health than any other treatments I tried.

The 5 Principles of Good Gut Health

As you probably realize by now, good gut health is more than any one single thing. Optimal gut health means taking good care of yourself and getting to the root cause of any digestive issues you may already have. Following these tips will put you on the path to healing.

You may have heard standard advice like "Just eat more fiber" or "Take a probiotic," and yet found that these tips have failed you so far. We are all incredibly unique, so standardized approaches aren't likely to meet your individual needs. By using a more tailored approach, you will help get to the root cause of your gut distress.

Good gut health strategies focus on five core principles: Remove, Replace, Repair, Repopulate, and Rebalance. I'll revisit these principles throughout the book.

1. **Remove.** This principle focuses on removing any triggers or sensitivities that may be altering your microbiome and causing inflammation in your body.

2. **Replace.** By replacing triggers with healthy foods and digestive compounds you may have been missing due to an imbalanced gut, you help your gut heal. This step can also include adding apple cider vinegar and enzymes or bile that have been missing due to an inflamed gut.

3. **Repair.** Adding high-nutrient foods and supplements when needed helps repair the gut lining. This is especially helpful for people who have had a diet full of processed foods in the past. Foods such as ginger and lemon and herbs such as mint can aid in repairing the gut as well.

4. **Repopulate.** Adding fermented foods, probiotics, and prebiotic foods to your diet helps repopulate your microbiome and restore gut health.

5. **Rebalance.** When you manage your stress, engage in meditation, exercise regularly, develop healthy sleep habits, and adopt healthy eating patterns, you help your gut rebalance.

Why a Holistic Approach Works

Why should you strive for a holistic approach? Research shows that being proactive in all areas of your health will help you heal most effectively. For example, you could eat a perfect diet, but if you are stressed out all the time, your healing will be partial. A holistic approach to gut health integrates many techniques to help you improve your overall health. It incorporates mind-body techniques, good sleep habits, nourishing foods, exercise, and some supplemental nutrients, when needed. But don't worry: Even if you aren't practicing all of these approaches at the same time, you will still experience benefits. When you make one positive change, it almost always promotes others.

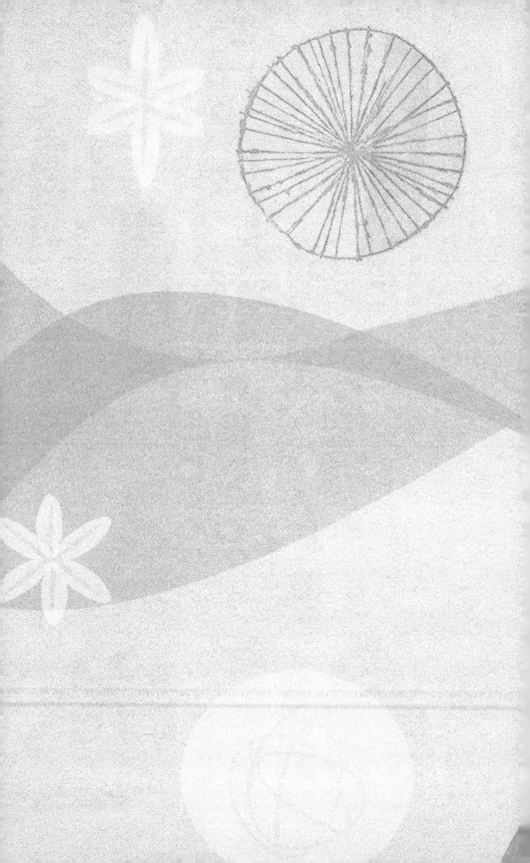

CHAPTER 2

Gut Check

This chapter will help you tune in to what good gut health feels like. You will also use a symptom tracker to identify symptoms of an imbalanced microbiome and learn how this imbalance can create disease in your body. Becoming aware of your body's signs and signals will help you respond to your body's needs more quickly and more fully. Many times, just a few adjustments in your daily habits can make a difference, but you'll also learn when it's time to seek help beyond the scope of this book.

Manifestations of Poor Gut Health

Because your microbiome is unique, the health issues related to it can present themselves in a variety of ways. In this section, you will learn about conditions that can be affected by gut health and how to identify their symptoms.

GI DISORDERS

Signs of a happy gut include feeling energized and having regular, easy bowel movements. A healthy gut is also free of heartburn, indigestion, belly pain, excess gas, and bloating. If you are experiencing a lack of energy, constipation, or any other gastrointestinal symptoms, begin by taking a look at your diet. Developing a holistic meal plan can help improve your microbiome, which will help alleviate your discomfort and ensure that the food you eat brings you energy and nourishment.

IRRITABLE BOWEL SYNDROME

The most common gut issue today is irritable bowel syndrome (IBS). There are no tests that can specifically diagnose IBS. Rather, by asking questions about your symptoms and ruling out other conditions, your doctor may conclude that you have IBS. Just because there is no specific test for IBS doesn't make it any less real or any less harmful to your health. Symptoms of IBS include abdominal pain, gas, bloating, diarrhea, and constipation.

INDIGESTION AND HEARTBURN

Common digestive concerns such as indigestion, heartburn, and reflux can be tricky to differentiate. Indigestion and heartburn have the same symptoms and can even be masking an underlying gallbladder issue. Symptoms of both include belching and gas, a feeling of discomfort after meals, a burning feeling in the stomach area or above, an acidic feeling, or nausea and vomiting. Often, the initial feeling will be that food is sitting in the stomach like a brick.

GALLBLADDER AND BILE ISSUES

Your gallbladder stores the bile made by your liver until your digestive system is ready to use it. If your gallbladder isn't working correctly, you can have a lot of discomfort after meals. Symptoms of gallbladder and bile issues can include pale-colored bowel movements, diarrhea, constipation, pain after meals, nausea and vomiting, or jaundice.

Gallbladder and bile issues can be sneaky, because they can flare up almost without notice. Over 20 million Americans have gallstones, and this number is, unfortunately, on the rise according to *World Journal of Gastroenterology*. The good news is that gallstones are largely thought to be preventable, and maintaining good gut health may help keep them at bay.

INFLAMMATORY BOWEL DISEASES

Inflammatory bowel diseases (IBD) include ulcerative colitis, Crohn's disease, and celiac disease. These conditions always present with inflammation in the large intestine and sometimes in the small intestine. Symptoms of IBD are sometimes obvious and sometimes not. For example, some people with celiac disease suffer for years without realizing that their digestive problems, pain, and depression are caused by gluten. With ulcerative colitis and Crohn's disease, people will often have diarrhea, constipation, weight loss, and pain that can be debilitating.

AUTOIMMUNE CONDITIONS

Autoimmune diseases are a group of over 100 diseases related to imbalances in the immune system. Autoimmune conditions have a genetic component, but they are also influenced by the microbiome, which means that improving your gut health can help improve and sometimes even reverse the symptoms of these debilitating conditions. Some examples of autoimmune diseases that can be improved by diet and microbiome changes are psoriasis, asthma, ankylosing spondylitis, eczema, lupus, and multiple sclerosis. Some studies have shown that an autoimmune protocol diet, which eliminates foods that cause sensitivities and inflammation and favors foods that restore microbiome health, may reduce fatigue and other symptoms of some of these conditions.

MENTAL HEALTH ISSUES

If your gut microbiome is off-kilter, your immune system sends a message to the brain that there is a threat. When your diet is always out of balance and your microbiome is sending regular alarm signals, your body feels like it's constantly in danger. Over the long term, the stress and inflammation that result from the body constantly being on high alert can contribute to anxiety and depression. Many studies link depression to an altered microbiome. At least 15 studies have been conducted to demonstrate that probiotics may help reduce symptoms of depression, and a systematic review of 21 studies in *General Psychiatry* concluded that improving the balance of the microbiome by using probiotics can help reduce anxiety symptoms.

Memory loss and dementia are also affected by your gut flora. Some studies show Alzheimer's disease has been linked to an altered microbiome and show that patients who take probiotics may suffer less severe memory loss. Consuming fermented yogurt, which is a rich source of probiotics, resulted in improved memory in two randomized, double-blind, placebo-controlled trials, even in healthy middle-age and older adults.

SKIN DISORDERS

Both the skin and the gut defend your body from pathogens—or harmful bacteria, viruses, and microorganisms—by acting as a protective barrier. But did you know your gut microbiome affects the microbiome that lives on your skin? It turns out that a healthy gut microbiome helps prevent and treat skin disorders, including acne, psoriasis, eczema, and even wrinkles. By bolstering your overall immune system, a healthy gut microbiome helps protect your skin, too.

HEART DISORDERS

According to the Centers for Disease Control and Prevention, more than 600,000 Americans die of heart disease each year. A lot of focus has been placed on investigating the link between saturated fats and heart disease, but emerging research suggests that a type of bacteria found in our microbiome is related to coronary artery disease, heart attacks, and even strokes. This relationship, however, does not necessarily mean that a gut imbalance is a direct cause of these conditions.

Probiotics can help reduce both systolic and diastolic blood pressure, and some clinical studies have found that probiotics help improve diabetes markers like high blood sugar and cholesterol ratios. These findings point to the fact that the microbiome has more impact on your heart health than was imagined 10 years ago.

GUT SCIENCE: LEAKY GUT SYNDROME

The father of medicine, Hippocrates, claimed that all diseases begin in the gut. He made that claim in the year 370 BCE. Now some of the most brilliant physicians in the world are proving him right through research.

Dr. Alessio Fasano first coined the term "leaky gut." While this term has remained controversial among some health-care providers, even Harvard Health has now embraced this as a real condition.

Remember your intestinal lining? Building block proteins help keep the tight junctions between cells in the intestinal lining closely knit together, which prevents unwanted pathogens from entering your bloodstream. There is a protein called zonulin, discovered by Dr. Fasano, that causes these cells to relax and open up. When your intestinal wall opens up, it essentially becomes "leaky," allowing substances into your bloodstream that don't belong there. Your body perceives these substances as a threat, which triggers an inflammatory response.

Elevated levels of zonulin are now linked to many diseases, such as depression, colitis, chronic fatigue, diabetes, obesity, type 1 diabetes, celiac disease, and multiple sclerosis. Common causes of increases in zonulin are thought to be gluten, ibuprofen, alcohol, imbalance in the microbiome, and food sensitivities. Keep in mind, however, that there are likely differences in how people respond to these substances, as well as how they respond to increases in zonulin.

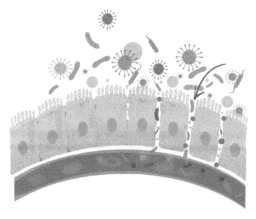

Identify Your Symptoms

By identifying your own unique symptoms and their triggers, you will be able to track your progress. Fill out the Symptom Tracker that follows by marking how often you're experiencing a specific symptom and writing down the food triggers you think might be causing it. You'll want to revisit this chart each week for three weeks. Each time, focus on how your gut is feeling, along with your overall mood, energy, and general health. Note if your symptoms change over time or are related to a specific time of day or situation. Finally, do a full-body scan and write down any other symptoms you are experiencing.

SYMPTOM TRACKER

SYMPTOM	NEVER	SOMETIMES*	FREQUENTLY**	FOOD TRIGGERS
Diarrhea (liquid stools that occur 2 to 3 times a day or more)				
Light-colored stools (tan or pasty-colored)				
Constipation (bowel movements are hard lumps, difficult to pass, and infrequent)				
Bowel urgency (difficulty making it to the bathroom in time)				
Bloating				
Belching				

*Sometimes (weekly or 2 to 3 times a week)   **Frequently (daily)

CONTINUED >>>

SYMPTOM	NEVER	SOMETIMES*	FREQUENTLY**	FOOD TRIGGERS
Flatulence				
Heartburn (belly pain, acid in the mouth, burning in the esophagus)				
Indigestion (discomfort after meals, sour feeling in the stomach)				
Nausea and/or vomiting				
Belly pain				
Brain fog				
Fatigue				
Anxious feelings in the gut				
Sadness				
Low energy				
Body aches and pains				
Cravings for sugar				
Other: _____				

*Sometimes (weekly or 2 to 3 times a week)   **Frequently (daily)

When to See a Doctor

There are times when you will need to seek the help of your doctor or health-care provider. For example, if you have nausea and vomiting daily or on a regular basis, make sure to seek help. Vomiting should occur very rarely if you are healthy, so it could be a sign of something more serious.

Additionally, if you develop blood in your stools or are vomiting blood for any reason, make sure to get medical help. Bloody stools or vomit are definitely a sign of something that needs to be urgently treated. Of course, if you are constipated, you can get hemorrhoids, which can cause some bleeding around the anus. While uncomfortable, this isn't always an urgent medical situation.

Heartburn, especially if it happens frequently or every day, can cause erosion of the esophagus and increase your risk of cancer. For this reason, it is important that your health-care provider rules out any sort of serious inflammation related to acid in the stomach or esophagus. More often than not, heartburn is related to your diet, but to be safe, always make sure to check in with your doctor if your symptoms don't improve with some healthy diet changes.

An imbalanced microbiome can make you sad, anxious, and forgetful. Following a holistic meal plan can improve your mood and energy, but if you start feeling worse for any reason, make sure to talk with your doctor.

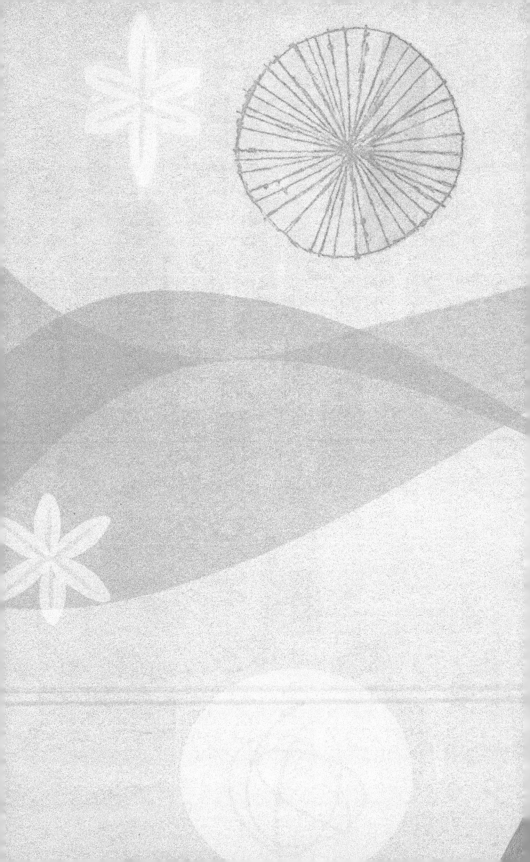

Part Two

The Holistic Path to Better Gut Health

CHAPTER 3

Nutrition

In this chapter, you will learn all about how food and nutrition affect your gut health. Then, on the practical side, you will learn food tips, including customized gut health dietary guidelines, some superstar gut foods, and the science of probiotics and prebiotics.

Food sensitivities can be a big trigger for gut issues, so you will learn about those here, too, as well as when to consider removing certain foods from your diet. The last section is dedicated to taking a critical look at supplements for gut health.

The Role of Nutrition in Gut Health

Without a doubt, the biggest thing you can do to improve your gut health is to be conscious about the foods you eat every day. If you are like most people, you are eating at least two or three times a day, which gives you many opportunities to nourish your intestinal cells and your microbiome with healthy, healing nutrients.

Your intestinal cells renew themselves every five days or so. This means that your diet can help your digestive health (or hurt it) in less than a week. Eating well will help support a healthy microbiome, reduce inflammation in your gut, and improve your overall health. While there are many specialized diets for gut health, such as GAPS and low-FODMAP, this book takes more of a gentle approach to long-term gut health. Just remember: You don't always have to be perfect. This plan is intended to be sustainable for you.

Dietary Guidelines

Later in this book, you will find a variety of recipes that help heal your gut, plus a two-week plan to get you started. First, there are some general nutritional guidelines you should strive to follow:

Eat fermented foods daily. Fermented foods such as sauerkraut, kimchi, yogurt, kombucha, and some types of pickles contain probiotics that support gut health. These foods are the primary sources of probiotics in your diet.

Don't skimp on protein. As part of a balanced diet, protein-rich foods offer the building blocks that your intestinal cells need for development and maintenance. Also, gut-healing minerals like zinc, magnesium, and selenium tag along with some protein-rich foods like seafood, fish, grass-finished meats, chicken, nuts, and even some legumes and grains. Legumes and grains, however, absolutely need to be soaked, (ideally) sprouted, and fermented for better gut health.

Eat the rainbow. By eating a variety of colorful produce every day, you will maximize the antioxidants in your diet, which can help reduce inflammation in your gut and your whole body. Get your blue from eggplant, currants, and blueberries; red from tomatoes and pomegranates; green from leafy vegetables and broccoli; orange from pumpkin, citrus, and peppers; and yellow from yellow beets, corn, and pineapple.

Remove common triggers for leaky gut. A common trigger for leaky gut is gluten, which can be found in grains such as wheat, barley, rye, and some oats (oats that are gluten-free are always labeled as such). Watch out for food additives and condiments, like soy sauce and malt vinegar, that have gluten, too. While you may not need to limit gluten forever, it is a good idea to go two to three weeks without it to see how you feel. Other possible triggers for leaky gut include ibuprofen, artificial sweeteners, alcohol, and processed sugars.

Have a helping of mushrooms regularly. Mushrooms contain beta-glucan, which provides prebiotics that help enrich the microbiome. People have eaten mushrooms for thousands of years for their medicinal effects. Research is now proving that mushrooms are indeed good medicine, especially for the gut.

Don't forget fiber-rich root vegetables, seeds, and nuts. Root vegetables such as sweet potatoes, turnips, and even potatoes are rich in fiber, antioxidants, and nutrients that may help improve your microbiome diversity. Seeds and nuts provide unique antioxidants that help protect your gut lining. They're more beneficial to the gut when soaked, sprouted, and cooked.

Consume some raw and cooked produce every day. Raw foods are rich in nutrients like vitamin C, antioxidants, and enzymes. In contrast, cooked foods provide more vitamin A and fermentable fibers, which are fibers that can be broken down into fuel for the intestinal cells.

Ditch processed foods as much as possible. Packaged and processed foods have begun to dominate the food shelves in grocery stores and restaurants, which is bad news for our microbiomes. Most processed foods are fraught with gut-busting ingredients like emulsifiers and additives, as well as an overabundance of sugar and simple carbs, all of which may negatively impact the microbiome.

Enjoy more spices and herbs in your dishes. One of the easiest ways to make your meals healthier and more enjoyable is by using generous amounts of a wide variety of spices and herbs (fresh or dried) in your dishes. They are great sources of antioxidants and gut-healing compounds. Enjoy them as herbal teas as well to boost your daily antioxidant intake and improve your mood.

Eat allium vegetables daily. Allium vegetables include onions, garlic, leeks, and scallions. These vegetables are beneficial to the microbiome and immune system due to their sulfur-containing compounds and prebiotics. These compounds help the immune system and may even fight digestive cancers.

12 Things Not to Do

While it's crucial to start tuning in to how you are feeling and how the things in your daily routine affect you, it's equally important to recognize habits that may be causing more harm than good in the long term.

1. **Don't rely on over-the-counter medications for having a regular bowel movement.** Using stool softeners, laxatives, or diarrhea medications regularly can cause dependence and result in loss of muscle and nerve response in the gut.

2. **Don't rely too much on heartburn medication.** Unless your doctor has deemed them required, these can ultimately deplete nutrients and worsen gut health. It's a good idea to have a detailed conversation with your doctor about the need for heartburn medication if you are currently on one, as research suggests that over 80 percent of heartburn medications prescribed are unnecessary.

3. **Don't forget to stay hydrated.** Dehydration makes both diarrhea and constipation worse and can cause headaches and fatigue.

4. **Don't forget to chew.** Chewing your food thoroughly at every meal is key for good digestive health.

5. **Don't focus on losing weight while healing your gut.** You need a good amount of all nutrients to make your body heal and function well.

6. **Don't take athletic supplements for performance.** These can lead to feelings of anxiety and gut distress due to their stimulants.

7. **Don't over-caffeinate.** This can cause anxious feelings in the stomach, poor sleep, nausea, and irritability.

8. **Don't embark on a bowel cleanse program.** Although some of these products can have healthy ingredients, a holistic meal plan should have enough fiber and foods that will keep you healthy and regular.

9. **Don't underestimate the time commitment.** Don't try the holistic plan for the first time when you are traveling or too busy to cook.

10. **Don't develop a fear of foods.** A holistic plan is meant to help you identify what works well, not create food phobias.

11. **Don't expect a uniform solution.** Remember that you are identifying what works best for you, not embarking on a restrictive diet for the rest of your life.

12. **Don't eat processed foods.** In a nutshell, you will want to avoid as much as possible anything that isn't in its whole or natural form.

GUT SCIENCE: PROBIOTICS AND PREBIOTICS

You've already heard about probiotics, but what exactly are they and how do they help you?

Probiotics

Probiotics are living microorganisms that positively affect your health. They include beneficial bacteria and yeasts that live in your microbiome, but they can also come from fermented foods such as sauerkraut, kimchi, kombucha, yogurt, aged cheeses, kefir, miso, tempeh, natto, fermented pickles, and fermented seeds and nuts. You can also buy probiotic supplements in capsules. Probiotics may help prevent leaky gut; improve immune function; reduce lactose intolerance, constipation, diarrhea, and irritable bowel syndrome; and improve your absorption of nutrients.

Starting slow is a good policy when introducing probiotics. For example, have 1 tablespoon of raw sauerkraut per day. If all is well after a few days, increase to 2 tablespoons. The same advice applies to supplements: Try a lower dose, such as 10 billion CFUs (colony-forming units) and increase based on your results.

Prebiotics

Prebiotics are fermentable fibers that serve as fuel for your resident probiotics and intestinal cells. Research shows that prebiotics may also help support a balanced pH level in the gut, improve the enteric nervous system's functions, and deter cancer growth. Foods that have a natural abundance of prebiotics include garlic, onions, asparagus, chia seeds, flaxseed, bananas, peaches, berries, leafy greens, mushrooms, jicama, sweet potatoes, seaweed, gluten-free oats, and chicory root.

Again, start slow. Add a little bit of new prebiotic food at a time so that your body has time to adapt. These are fiber-rich foods, so if your body is not used to them, you can get a significant amount of gas and bloating unless you slowly increase them over time.

What to Eat and What to Avoid

The following list is meant to help guide you on your journey to better gut health through nutrition. For all the foods listed here, it is best to choose organic whenever possible in all categories. This is because nonorganic foods are often sprayed with chemicals that may impair your microbiome. If you can't find or can't afford organic vegetables, try to choose unsprayed. I also recommend sprouting all legumes (see page 132), soaking nuts (see page 108), and fermenting whole grains (see page 110) at home whenever possible for easier digestion and to reap maximum nutritional benefits. Fermented foods that you can buy in the supermarket are noted for easy reference.

FOODS TO ENJOY

DAIRY AND EGGS

Aged cheeses (fermented)

Buttermilk (fermented)

Cultured sour cream (fermented)

Dairy and nondairy yogurt (fermented)

Eggs

Kefir (fermented)

MEAT AND POULTRY

Chicken

Grass-finished beef

Turkey

Wild game

SEAFOOD

Anchovies

Clams

Cod

Crab

Haddock

Kipper snacks

Light tuna

Lobster

Mackerel

Mussels

Sardines

Shrimp

Snapper

Trout

Wild-caught salmon

FRUITS

Fermented fruits

Fresh papaya (eaten with meals)

Fresh pineapple (eaten with meals)

Lemon (fresh or fermented, eaten with meals)

Lime (eaten with meals)

Olives

VEGETABLES

Artichoke

Arugula

Asparagus

Avocado

Bean sprouts

Beets, greens and root

Broccoli

Broccoli sprouts

Brussels sprouts

Cabbage

Carrots

Cauliflower

Celery

Corn

Cucumbers

Fennel

Fermented vegetables

Fresh and dried herbs

Garlic

Green beans

Jalapeños

Jicama

Kale

Leeks

Mushrooms

Onions

Peas

Pumpkin

Radishes

Rutabagas

Scallions

Spinach

Sweet Potatoes

Turnips

Tomatillos

Tomatoes

Watercress

Winter squash

Zucchini

LEGUMES

Miso (fermented)

Natto (fermented)

Soaked beans

Tempeh (fermented)

NUTS AND SEEDS

Chia seeds

Flaxseed

Hemp seeds

Nut butters

Nuts

Pumpkin seeds

Sunflower seeds

GRAINS AND FLOURS

Amaranth

Brown rice (fermented)

Coconut flour

Soaked quinoa

FATS

Avocado oil

Coconut oil

Extra-virgin olive oil

CONDIMENTS

Fermented pickles

Kimchi (fermented)

Sauerkraut (fermented)

Tamari

Unfiltered apple cider vinegar (fermented)

BEVERAGES

Filtered water

Herbal teas

Kombucha (fermented)

Lemon water

FOODS TO EAT IN MODERATION

DAIRY

Try to limit to 1 serving per day.

Butter

Cream

Cream cheese

Fresh cheeses, like mozzarella

Milk

FRUITS

Limit to 2 to 3½ cups fresh or ½ cup dried per day, unless otherwise noted.

Apples

Apricots

Bananas

Blackberries (1 cup)

Blueberries (1 cup)

Cherries

Dates (¼ cup)

Figs, dried (¼ cup)

Figs, fresh

Grapefruit

Grapes

Kiwi

Melons (1½ cups)

Oranges

Peaches

Plums

Pomegranate

Raspberries (1 cup)

Raisins (¼ cup)

Watermelon (1½ cups)

VEGETABLES

Limit to 1 cup (cooked) per day.

Cassava root

Potatoes (white)

Tiger nuts

LEGUMES

Limit to 1 cup (cooked) total per day.

Black beans

Black-eyed peas

Chickpeas

Edamame

Kidney beans

Lentils

Lima beans

Mung beans

Navy beans

Pinto beans

Tofu

GRAINS AND FLOURS

Limit to ½ cup (dry) or 1 cup (cooked) per day.

Amaranth

Brown rice

Buckwheat

Cornmeal (non-GMO)

Gluten-free oats

Millet

Sorghum

Teff

Whole-grain all-purpose gluten-free flour

BEVERAGES

Limit to 1 cup coffee or tea per day and 1 (12-ounce) can carbonated water.

Black tea

Carbonated water (club soda, sparkling water, or flavored sparkling water)

Coffee

Green tea

SWEETENERS

Limit to 1 tablespoon per day of honey and maple syrup and 1 teaspoon of stevia and monk fruit.

Monk fruit sweetener

Raw honey

Real maple syrup

Stevia

FOODS TO AVOID

DAIRY

American cheese

Cheese spreads

MEAT AND POULTRY

If you can find uncured and all-natural versions, you can have these foods. Just be sure to limit it to small amounts due to their high sodium content (1 to 2 ounces).

Bacon

Deli meats

Hot dogs

Luncheon meats

Pepperoni

Sausages

Summer sausage

SEAFOOD

These fish are high in mercury.

Ahi tuna

Albacore tuna

Bigeye tuna

King mackerel

Marlin

Orange roughy

Shark

Swordfish

Tilefish

GRAINS AND FLOURS

Gluten hides in many packaged foods. Make sure to read ingredient lists and avoid products that say "Contains wheat."

Barley

Breads made with barley, rye, or wheat

Cookies, crackers, desserts, muffins, pastries, and snacks made with wheat flour

Soups and stews thickened with wheat flour roux

Wheat and wheat flour

Wheat-based pastas

FATS

Canola oil

Corn oil

Hydrogenated and partially hydrogenated oils

Light olive oil

Palm oil

Peanut oil

Refined coconut oil

Soybean oil

Sunflower oil

Vegetable oils

CONDIMENTS

Barbecue sauce

Bottled salad dressings

Malt vinegar

Soy sauce

BEVERAGES

Alcohol seltzers

Beer

Energy drinks

Hard liquor

Juices

Lemonade (unless made with raw honey)

Soda (both regular and diet)

Sports drinks

Wine

SWEETENERS

Acesulfame-K

Aspartame

Erythritol

High-fructose corn syrup

Maltitol

Sorbitol

Splenda

Sucralose

Sugar

Xylitol

Candy

Chips

Fast foods

Frozen desserts

Packaged cake and cookie mixes

Restaurant foods with processed grains or meats (pasta dishes, breads, sandwiches)

5 GUT-HEALING SUPERSTAR FOODS

There is strong research to support the digestive benefits of these five gut-healing foods, and I've found that most of my clients reap the benefits from these foods very quickly. By incorporating these superstars regularly in your diet, you will be jump-starting the Repair and Rebalance steps of the 5 Principles of Good Gut Health (see page 8).

1. **Ginger.** Fresh ginger root is full of antioxidants that support gut health, and a study showed it may also enhance your absorption of nutrients. It contains enzymes that help improve the digestive process and reduce nausea. This may be because it improves the muscle movements of the intestine. In my clinical experience, it's also effective for heartburn.

2. **Raw sauerkraut.** Perhaps the biggest gut-healing superstar of all, a study in the journal *PLoS One* found that raw sauerkraut is teeming with as many as 114 different strains of probiotics. By helping immune function in the gut, sauerkraut and other fermented vegetables may also ease autoimmune-related digestive concerns, such as gastritis and colitis.

3. **Mushrooms.** Culinary mushrooms are good for digestion because they are rich in prebiotic fibers and gut-healing minerals like selenium and zinc. Mushrooms also enhance gut immunity by boosting T-cell counts and improving the diversity of the microbiome. Research shows that shiitake mushrooms may help fight gastric cancers, too.

CONTINUED >>>

4. **Broccoli sprouts.** Rich in an antioxidant compound called sulforaphane, broccoli sprouts can help reduce constipation and may help remove toxins from the body. Broccoli sprouts may also reduce colitis, diabetes, and cancer risk. If you can't find broccoli sprouts, eating raw broccoli can help, but the concentration of sulforaphane it contains is lower.

5. **Wild sardines.** Wild sardines are rich in minerals, vitamins, protein, and omega-3 fatty acids, all of which are important for maintaining a healthy intestinal lining. Omega-3s may also decrease inflammatory bowel diseases. Additionally, a small study found that wild sardines increased the health of the microbiome in people with diabetes. Don't like sardines? Try salmon, shrimp, or trout.

Navigating Food Sensitivities

Digestive problems often boil down to food sensitivities and allergies. Eliminating foods that cause sensitivities can greatly benefit your digestion and your overall health. Navigating food sensitivities is part of the Remove principle of good gut health (see page 8).

Ultimately, the best way to know if you are sensitive to foods is to do a full elimination diet. This entails eliminating foods that commonly cause sensitivities and allergies for three to four weeks and then reintroducing them one at time to discover your triggers. The foods that most commonly cause sensitivities are gluten, dairy, soy, corn, eggs, peanuts, tree nuts, and seafood. On an elimination diet, you will also be encouraged to eat whole foods and discouraged from eating processed foods.

Other food sensitivities include histamine intolerance and nightshade sensitivity. Histamines can come from foods such as avocados, alcohol, spinach, citrus, beans, and tomatoes, and people with nightshade sensitivities should avoid tomatoes, potatoes, eggplant, gooseberries, and peppers. While these foods are not the first line of elimination to try, it could be worth doing if other elimination diets don't identify what is causing your digestive distress.

Elimination diets can prove more useful and direct than allergy or sensitivity tests. While you can do both, allergy and sensitivity tests can fail to catch triggers, so the best way to fully know if you are sensitive to a food is to use the elimination process.

The good news is that for people with sensitivities, there are a lot of good substitutions available in supermarkets today. For example, people with a dairy sensitivity or allergy will find a lot of good dairy-free alternatives like coconut- or almond-based based yogurts, rice milk, oat milk, coconut milk, and dairy-free cheeses. For a gluten intolerance or wheat allergy, substitutions include coconut-, almond-, and rice-based flours, as well as gluten-free crackers, pizza crusts, and pastas, to name a few.

Are Supplements Necessary?

Supplements can do exactly what their name suggests: supplement your diet. They are part of the Repair principle of good gut health (see page 8). Whether supplements help you is dependent on where you are in your health journey and what your symptoms are. Read the descriptions of the supplements in this section to determine if any may help alleviate some of the symptoms you identified in the Symptom Tracker (see page 17). Always try to find high-quality brands that have Good Manufacturing Practices (GMP) and follow dosing suggestions on the label unless otherwise advised by your doctor.

VITAMIN D

Humans get most of their vitamin D from the sun. Yet as many as 29 percent of Americans are deficient and 41 percent are insufficient in this critical nutrient. In ideal amounts, vitamin D has antimicrobial effects, helps protect the epithelial lining, reduces inflammation, and keeps the microbiome in better balance.

MAGNESIUM

Low magnesium can reduce your microbiome diversity and make you constipated. Stomach acid medications can cause poor absorption of magnesium and other minerals. It can take several months of supplementation to get your body back to a normal magnesium balance.

BILE

People with long-term diarrhea or those who have had their gallbladder removed are at risk for low bile, reducing their ability to absorb fat and fat-soluble vitamins. A telltale sign of low bile is a pale-colored stool. In my experience, low bile symptoms improve fairly quickly after taking bile supplements combined with digestive enzymes.

ENZYMES

Digestive enzymes help break down foods so you can absorb their nutrients. One enzyme you may be familiar with is lactase (sold as Lactaid). *Current Drugs and Metabolism* suggests that enzyme supplements hold a lot of potential for benefiting digestive health. For my clients, gas and bloating are often reduced when they take digestive enzymes with meals.

GLUTAMINE

If you have inflammation in your gut due to a poor diet or inflammatory bowel disease, a supplement that may be useful in the short term is glutamine. Normally, our bodies make enough glutamine, but under stressful conditions, supplemental glutamine may help reduce leaky gut.

ZINC

Potential causes of zinc deficiency include diarrhea, a restrictive diet, a diet of processed foods, or inflammation. A short-term supplemental regimen of zinc can be especially helpful if you have been dealing with diarrhea, as it reduces inflammation and helps improve gut barrier function.

A GUT FEELING

Gut health can seem confusing, but with a little investigative work, the effects of food and nutrition on gut health become quite clear. Here's a story from a client of mine:

> "My quest for gut health began as a search to end an unexplained abdominal pain. I didn't know it was gut health I was reaching for. Traditional medicine had provided caring professionals who, using every conceivable tool available to them, could find no explanation and had declared me remarkably healthy. But I still had this inexplicable pain. Unrealized by me at the time, I was also experiencing so many other ongoing symptoms that were a signal to an unhealthy gut and microbiome.
>
> When I took an over-the-counter histamine-blocking pill after mistakenly eating some gluten, I realized it stopped the abdominal pain.
>
> So the journey began, with my RD's leadership, to embrace a low histamine diet to see if I could heal entirely. I had never considered that a possibility, but now I do. Aside from not having any abdominal pain anymore, my head is already so much clearer, a side effect of a healthy gut I didn't know I was missing. I'm happier, have more energy, and dive into projects instead of procrastinating. I had no idea my gut had anything to do with any of this. My journey to better gut health has been very rewarding and has literally changed my life."

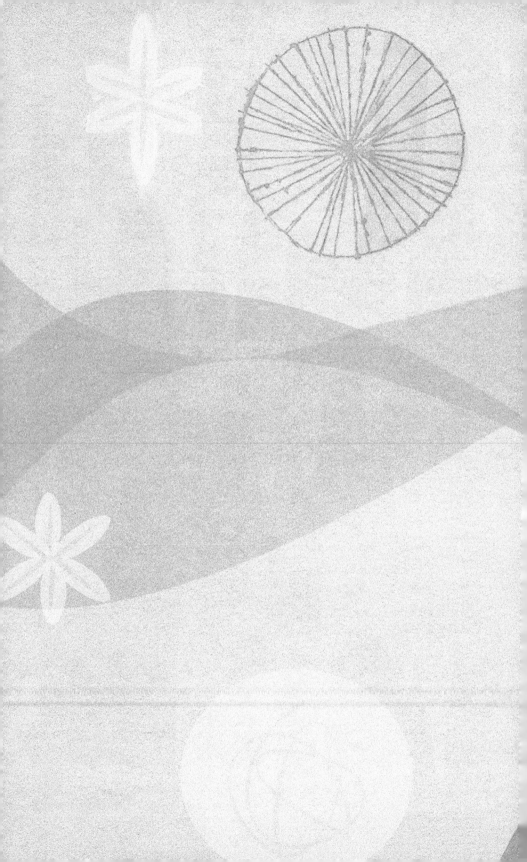

CHAPTER 4

Exercise and Physical Health

In this chapter, you'll learn about the benefits of exercise for your gut health, specifically how it impacts your metabolism, circulation, endorphins, microbiome, motility, and stress hormones. You'll learn how different types of exercise affect your gut in different ways, as well as some easy and practical tips to make exercise more enjoyable and some of the best yoga poses for digestion.

Other factors that affect your gut health are also discussed here, including how sunlight affects your gut, the role of sleep for digestive health, and how elimination diets and fasting may fit into your gut-healing routines.

The Role of Exercise in Gut Health

Regular exercise benefits more than just your muscular system and your heart. You're boosting all aspects of your digestive health, too. Exercise is part of the Rebalance principle of the 5 Principles of Good Gut Health (see page 8) because it restores healthy gut muscle movements, supports a healthy metabolism, helps maintain your hormone balance, improves neurotransmitters, and more. Exercise may even help increase the diversity of healthy bacteria in your gut while reducing symptoms of digestive diseases. Symptoms of irritable bowel disease, constipation, gallbladder diseases, and inflammatory bowel diseases all seem to be alleviated by exercise. Let's dig into some of the effects of exercise on your gut health.

METABOLISM

The metabolism centers of your cells, even in your gut, are your mitochondria. When you exercise, you increase the number of mitochondria and the efficiency of nutrient metabolism by them, meaning more nutrients are available to your gut. Both aerobic and strength-training exercises improve the function of mitochondria. Overall, by increasing your metabolism through exercise, you increase your quantity of mitochondria and your ability to absorb nutrients from your food, resulting in increased energy.

CIRCULATION

When you exercise, your heart pumps harder, your blood vessels receive more oxygen, your carbon dioxide exchange is increased, and your digestive tract receives more blood flow. This increased blood circulation during exercise is important because it facilitates the exchange of nutrients, oxygen, and carbon dioxide between the gut and your cardiovascular system. Added benefits to the circulatory system from exercise include reduced arterial stress, reduced toxins, reduced inflammation, and a healthier microbiome.

ENDORPHINS

By exercising regularly, you will also dampen the effects of chronic stress and enjoy an increase in "happy" neurotransmitters called endorphins. Endorphins contribute to what some people call a "runner's high." But you don't have to do intense exercise like running to trigger a surge in endorphins and other positive neurotransmitters. The important part of exercise is that you do it regularly and that you do something you enjoy. What does all of this have to do with gut health? Simply put, when your mood improves, so does your gut health.

STRESS HORMONES

Stress, whether short-term or chronic, can affect your digestive system. This is because fear hormones, like adrenaline and cortisol, reduce digestive function. Think of it like this: If you are running from a tiger, your body isn't prioritizing the digestion of your sandwich. It is prioritizing running fast! While most people aren't running from tigers these days, the stress hormones that surge daily due to our fast-paced lifestyles disrupt normal digestion unless you learn to manage your stress. Exercise has a net effect of reducing stress hormones in your body, which helps your body digest food better and supports a balanced microbiome.

MOTILITY

A healthy digestive tract has healthy motility, with the movements of the intestinal muscles being referred to as peristalsis. Exercise naturally stimulates these movements via enteric nervous system activation. By stimulating peristalsis and stomach emptying, exercise can help alleviate symptoms of heartburn and indigestion. Not all exercise is running or lifting weights; motility can be improved simply by doing breathing exercises.

Know Your Exercises

The World Health Organization recommends that people get a minimum of 150 minutes of moderate exercise per week or around 20 minutes per day. There are four key categories of exercise—aerobic, strength-building, flexibility, and breathing—but many types of exercise involve more than one category. Yoga is an especially good multi-category exercise, and even something like gardening can be both aerobic and strength-building.

AEROBIC

You don't have to be an elite athlete to enjoy the gut health benefits of aerobic exercise. Research shows that women who were previously sedentary gain beneficial gut bacteria after just seven days of increased aerobic exercise. These women increased both the amount and diversity of their healthy bacteria diversity in this short time.

Aerobic exercise is any exercise that gets your heart rate up from resting and includes brisk walking, running, swimming, hiking, cycling, and even gardening, dancing in your living room, and vigorous housework! (In the case of gardening, you reap additional benefits due to breathing in healthy microbes present in the soil and air.)

STRENGTH-BUILDING

While aerobic exercise is good for everyone, not all people are cut out to be endurance athletes. Some people are better power athletes, favoring the short bursts of strength used in exercises like squats, push-ups, abdominal exercises, and gardening. In addition to increasing muscle strength, these exercises can positively affect your metabolism and give you more energy.

Most research up to now has focused on how aerobic exercise benefits the microbiome, but anyone who has done strength exercises also knows that their heart rate increases while doing them. Odds are you gain the same gut benefits from lifting weights or doing resistance exercises as you do from cardio, but more research is needed to confirm this.

FLEXIBILITY

Exercises focused on flexibility are just as important as aerobic or strength workouts, yet there's been less research focused on them. Basic stretching helps with flexibility, as does yoga, or mind-body-breath integration with stretching, which has been used for thousands of years for its gut health benefits, especially its help in reducing symptoms of irritable bowel syndrome. In addition to flexibility and improved breath, yoga also builds strength. It's the ultimate holistic exercise!

BREATHING

You might not be thinking of breathing as an exercise, but slow, intentional breathing from the diaphragm, also known as belly breathing, can benefit just about every aspect of digestive function, especially motility. Slowly breathing in and out through your nose can also decrease stress hormones and get your body out of fight-or-flight mode.

You can focus on improving your breath by practicing long, slow exhales through your nose when you are at rest or during light activity like yoga and walking. By breathing through the nose, the breath is more controlled and can even make more vigorous exercise easier. Other ways to improve breath for digestive benefits include singing, humming, and even gargling. These may seem a little silly, but by stimulating the vagus nerve, these activities may improve your digestive muscle movements.

6 Essential Exercise Tips

1. **Make exercise a habit.** All habits can take a while to become part of your routine, so make sure to develop an exercise schedule. Set your alarm clock to get up from your desk at work or make plans with a buddy to go exercise after work every week. At work, take the stairs instead of the elevator or plan walking meetings.

2. **Find exercises that you enjoy.** You will be so much more likely to exercise if you find activities that you enjoy. Any little way you can fit in some more activity is great. Stretch while you are watching your favorite show in the evening. Some of my clients' most rewarding exercises to do are gardening or rearranging furniture.

3. **Listen to your body.** You will be much more likely to keep exercising if you listen to your body and only push yourself to a manageable level of exertion. This is especially important when you are beginning a new kind of exercise. If you overdo it and strain yourself, you can do more harm than good.

4. **Gradually increase your exercise.** If you gradually increase your time and exertion level, you will be less likely to injure yourself and more likely to stick to your exercise plan.

5. **Vary your exercise routine.** Your body will benefit more if you vary your routine between aerobic, strength, flexibility, and breath training. For example, alternate between hiking, yoga, gardening, dancing, and martial arts.

6. **Days off are important, too.** You don't have to hit it hard every day. Your body will need recovery days to help restore balance. You might want to have a day of the week dedicated to an easy stroll around your neighborhood as a rest day.

Using Yoga to Heal Your Gut

Yoga is a wonderful form of exercise that you can do almost anywhere, and it's great for almost every age, body type, and fitness level. Here are some yoga poses to try that can help your digestive tract.

CHILD'S POSE

Child's pose is a very natural position for the body. It slightly compresses the digestive organs, which helps stimulate digestive function when you are done. First, kneel on the floor with your toes touching together. Position your knees as wide as your hips or wider. Lay your body down between your thighs and stretch your arms out in front of your body, getting a gentle and relaxing stretch. Make sure to take slow, long breaths through your nose, making an ocean sound with your breath if you can. Hold this stretch for about one minute.

SUPINE TWIST

Supine twist helps stretch the large intestine, which can help with bowel regularity. Lie on your back with your legs stretched out naturally. Bring your right knee over your left to feel a gentle stretch through your lower back. Extend your right arm out to the right and try to keep your right shoulder on the ground. You can place your left hand over your right knee to give the stretch a little extra twist if you desire. Keep your breaths long and slow. Hold for about one minute and then repeat on the left side.

BRIDGE POSE

Bridge pose stretches the back and helps compress the digestive tract, increasing blood supply to both areas. Lie on your back and bring your feet in close toward your buttocks. Slowly lift your torso off the ground in a gentle motion and hold your torso up, pressing your feet into the ground. Bring your arms straight under your body if you can, and feel free to clasp your hands together. This should feel like a good back and abdomen stretch. Breathe slowly for at least 10 breath cycles.

REVOLVED CHAIR TWIST

This pose helps release a rush of fresh blood into your digestive system when you are done. Revolved chair twist begins by standing up straight while breathing slowly and easily, making oceanic breath sounds if you can throughout. Next sit back as if you were going to sit in a chair, making sure your knees don't come in front of your toes. Bring your hands together at your heart, pressing them together.

Once you feel comfortable, slowly bring your right elbow to the outside of your left knee. Using your elbow as leverage, give your torso a little extra stretch. Hold for several breath cycles. Come back to standing slowly just as you came into the pose. Repeat this sequence, this time bringing your left elbow to the outside of your right knee.

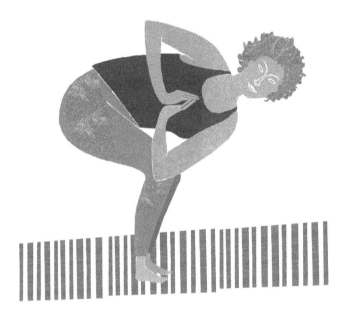

What Else Affects Gut Health?

Many of your daily habits affect your gut health. This section gives you an overview of how simple things like getting some sun, quality sleep, and meditating can improve your gut health, as well as how to time your meals ideally and how to eliminate food sensitivities.

SUNLIGHT

When you get enough natural sunlight, you will sleep better, have a healthier microbiome, and have fewer aches and pains because you will have more natural vitamin D in your body. Vitamin D is critical for gut health and helps your immune cells function correctly.

Midday sun is best for boosting your vitamin D levels. Keep in mind that if you are in a car or behind a window, you will not get the same benefits because the rays are refracted by the glass or plastic.

Sunblock also prevents you from getting the benefits from sunlight. However, it is important to remember that excessive sun exposure is linked to skin cancer, so avoid sunburn and lengthy sessions in the sun. Cover up with long sleeves and long pants and wear a hat if you are out for extended periods.

A very important part of knowing if you have enough vitamin D for your gut health is to have your doctor check your vitamin D levels, preferably twice a year. If you are like most people, you may need to complement your sun exposure with vitamin D supplements.

SLEEP

A healthy sleep cycle dictates much of your body's health, including your digestive health. One or two nights of sleep deprivation can throw your gut immune function into a tailspin. You can help your sleep quality and duration by getting daytime sunlight, making sure your room is dark before you go to bed, and putting away electronic devices at least 30 minutes before going to sleep.

Other simple tips for improving your sleep quality are to breathe slowly for several breath cycles throughout the day, and make sure to eat your last meal several hours before you go to sleep so you can digest your food well and avoid heartburn. Cut off the caffeine as early in the day as you can. I try to make sure I'm done with my tea or coffee by 11 a.m. Research shows that most people's sleep suffers if they have caffeine after 2 p.m.

FASTING

We all fast when we sleep, but the number of hours we do so varies from person to person. By intentionally extending the nighttime fast, you can reap some gut health benefits. This is because fasting helps reduce inflammation. If you stop eating for the day at 6 p.m., for example, you will be less likely to wake up during the night due to indigestion.

Start with fasting for 12 hours and work your way up to 16 hours per day if you can. Not only do people who fast have healthier digestive health, they may lower their cancer and heart disease risk, too. Bear in mind that if you have diabetes, are pregnant, or have other medical conditions, you should talk to your doctor before extending your fast. Consuming any foods or liquids with calories will end the fast, so make sure that you only have water during the fasting hours. Some people do more extreme fasting, such as water fasts or juice fasts. I recommend that you only do these under the close supervision of your doctor.

MEDITATING

Meditating is good for all aspects of wellness, including digestive health, and can be done by anyone. I'll admit that meditation was challenging for me at first and is challenging for many people, but there are some tools available that can be very helpful as you get started.

One type of meditation is guided self-hypnosis, also known as guided meditation. Hypnosis isn't as scary as some people think. Rather it is your own mind bringing itself into a deeply relaxed state. We all do meditation every day, whether we know it or not: The proof that you do is that you fall asleep. Meditation is simply the dreamy, wandering state your brain is in as it begins to relax.

You can find some good guided meditation and guided self-hypnosis videos on YouTube. I recommend Michael Sealey's guided meditation and sleep hypnosis videos. If you still are struggling to meditate, consider seeking the help of a clinical hypnotherapist or licensed counselor.

A GUT FEELING

Exercise makes your gut feel better in so many tangible ways. The beauty of exercise is that even a little bit can help how your gut is feeling. In my experience, even a small amount helps improve people's moods, and this is no coincidence.

A client of mine, Jennifer, explains what exercise means for her own gut health. "First, exercise keeps me regular. If I'm feeling bloated, I go out for a walk and it helps reduce the belly discomfort, too. Another big reason I exercise is that it reduces my stress. Stress is really constipating for me, so exercise is a must to prevent this. I think that my stress is better when I exercise because it's helping my gut function better.

The more routine I am with my exercise, the better I feel, because then I can enjoy my exercise more and I get more out of it. I don't feel as good when I don't have my exercise routine in place. I try to do things I love like walking, biking, and yoga, and I rotate these because they are equally fun for me."

Establishing a regular routine and doing exercises you love are the best ways to get the most from your exercise. Even if the routine feels a bit like a chore at first, your body may begin to crave the happy belly feelings that you get when you exercise.

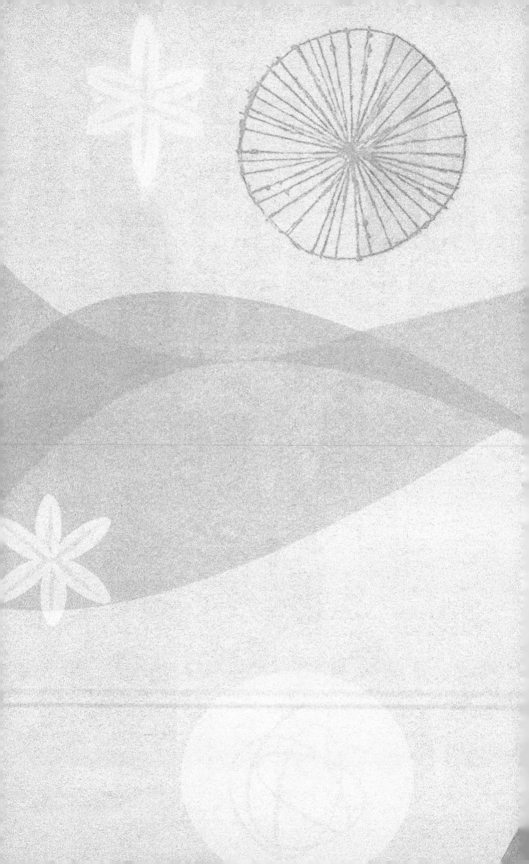

CHAPTER 5

Mental Health

In this chapter, you will learn about the deep connections between your mental health and your gut health. You'll find some simple tips to help manage stress, anxiety, and depression that you can do at home or at work. You will also learn about your adrenal function and whether "adrenal fatigue" is real.

Your chances of developing anxiety and depression are exceedingly high if you live in the United States, so learning to recognize, reduce, and manage the symptoms of these conditions is critical to maintaining your overall well-being. Meditation is an essential component of a healthy mind and gut, so I will also walk you through three easy meditation routines. I will also describe when to seek more help, if needed.

How Anxiety Affects Your Gut

When you are stressed, odds are you feel it in your gut. It is important to know that "stress" and "anxiety" are other words for fear. Remember the fear of being chased by a tiger? In today's world, rather than a tiger, you might be afraid of performing poorly at work, not getting to work on time due to traffic or other problems, tense political situations, money problems, tensions in a relationship, or any number of other daily stressors. According to the American Institute of Stress, 77 percent of Americans experience stress on a regular basis. There is no way that humans are equipped to handle that much stress and still be healthy.

Daily feelings of stress disrupt your digestion in many ways. Your body puts its efforts toward creating stress hormones like cortisol. High levels of cortisol, which is created in your adrenal glands, shut down normal functioning of your digestive tract. While you need cortisol in your body to fight an infection (or run from a tiger), having a tank full of cortisol every day is very damaging to your gut health and your overall health.

Stress can alter your microbiome, and chronic stress impairs your microbiome and your immune function. Stress and anxiety make you more likely to suffer from digestive concerns, such as ulcers, gallstones, inflammatory bowel disease, irritable bowel disease, heartburn, indigestion, diarrhea, and constipation. As you have learned, these problems are compounded by a reduced ability to absorb nutrients and by a poor microbiome generating additional stress signals.

When you are stressed out, you are also more prone to a leaky gut, because your healthy microbiome is compromised. You have less blood flow to the digestive tract, fewer healthy bacteria to nourish the lining, decreased production of the mucus lining, more inflammation, and ultimately, fewer protective immune cells.

If you add stress eating (which often means junk food) into the mix, you'll make your leaky gut worse because you're depriving your digestive tract of nutrients, fueling bad bacteria, increasing inflammation and toxins, and altering bile flow. The result: even worse belly issues and malaise.

By now, you may be feeling stressed out about being stressed out. That is not my goal; rather, my goal is to help you become aware of the need to better manage daily stressors. For example, might there be a more relaxing way to get to work? Can you listen to relaxing music or an interesting podcast during your commute? The next section is dedicated to practical advice for reducing stress.

GUT SCIENCE: IS "ADRENAL FATIGUE" A REAL THING?

The adrenal glands produce stress hormones like cortisol and adrenaline, as well as sex hormones like testosterone and estrogen. Some health professionals have coined the term "adrenal fatigue" for people who have been stressed out for so long that their bodies aren't making adequate levels of hormones like cortisol anymore. The resulting symptoms can include fatigue, hopelessness, low blood pressure, low sex drive, feeling cold, restlessness, and craving snacks.

Whether or not adrenal fatigue truly exists is hotly debated. Some contend that fatigue and the other symptoms are not caused by low cortisol at all but can be caused by stress-induced inflammation in the body. To me, it seems a matter of semantics: We know stress is bad for the body and severe stress is associated with low cortisol, as is the case with post-traumatic stress disorder. If low cortisol is due to adrenal fatigue or some other related factor, it doesn't really matter. You will benefit by reducing stress no matter what, because stress causes damage and inflammation in the whole body, including the adrenal glands.

Trauma, whether physical or mental, results in alterations in the gut microbiome. Taking steps to nurture your microbiome by reducing stress, eating fermented foods, enjoying lots of gut-healthy foods, taking time for self-care, and getting good sleep will help ensure that you never have to worry about getting adrenal fatigue at all.

5 Ways to Reduce Stress

Stress management is critical for good gut health and overall well-being. Here are five healthy ways to reduce stress in your life.

If you have severe anxiety or experience panic attacks, make sure to contact your doctor or therapist. Sometimes getting a good handle on stress requires some personalized help.

1. **Listen to music.** Playing some of your favorite relaxing music can alleviate stress and help reduce depression and anxiety. Listening to music that you love also decreases your stress response, which has a positive impact on your gut; in contrast, noise pollution may impair a healthy gut. In this case, you may consider getting noise-canceling headphones or finding a quiet place to listen. The type of music that reduces stress will be unique to you, so choose what speaks to you in the moment.

2. **Try essential oils.** Essential oils are concentrated plant extracts that may help ease feelings of anxiety. Your sense of smell is directly connected to the limbic system in the brain, so when you smell certain plant compounds like essential oils, it may slow down the release of cortisol. Diffuse a little bit of essential oil anytime you need a little stress relief, but keep in mind a little goes a long way. Make sure to get pure, therapeutic brands whenever possible and do not diffuse any plant oils to which you may be sensitive.

3. **Spend time with friends, family, or a pet.** This tip seems obvious, but sometimes you may forget to connect with the people around you. Isolation is a big stress trigger for many people, so calling a friend or family member or making a plan to get together can help. And remember, your pet is always there for you, too. You can tell them pretty much anything, and they won't judge!

4. **Dig in the dirt.** You don't have to have a giant yard to get the benefit of gardening and having plants; get some pots and some potting soil for your house or yard and find out how soothing it can be to grow things both inside and outside your home. Connecting with the earth and living plants helps reduce stress and improve your microbiome. If you're not able to have a garden

or houseplants, visit public gardens or open spaces whenever you can.

5. **Keep a journal.** Brains sometimes have a hard time shutting off because they are a library of past, present, and future stressors. By writing down your thoughts and your stressors, you'll be able to start to see patterns in your life that may not be serving you well. Then you can focus on simple steps to address your specific issues and habits. Sometimes the writing process itself, whether on paper or on the computer, can be relaxing. No need to worry about grammar or spelling—just write it all down and remember that no one is going to critique this journal. It is yours alone.

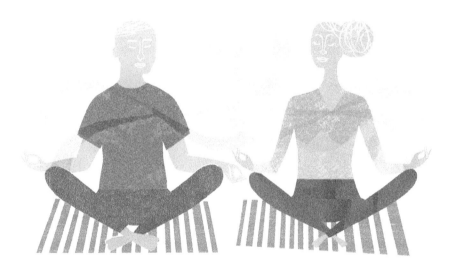

How Depression Affects Your Gut

The National Institute of Mental Health estimates that over 16 million Americans suffer from depression each year and that there is about a 1 in 5 chance that a person may experience major depression in their lifetime. Just like stress, depression gets communicated back and forth between your gut and your brain. For example, people who have depression tend to also have constipation and other digestive issues, and people who tend to be constipated have higher chances of feeling depressed. Depression can also cause increased cramping or belly pain. Up to 34 percent of people with depression experience either increased belly pain or irritable bowel syndrome.

Many experts in the field of psychiatry are now proposing that depression is related to an imbalance in the immune system, which is rooted in the gut microbiome. So truly, the health of your gut microbiome dictates your overall health and happiness.

Depression can be caused by other factors, too, so it is important to look at your health, personal habits, symptoms, and events in your life through a holistic lens. For example, grief, loss, physical or emotional abuse, drugs, alcohol, and serious illnesses can all cause depression. Addressing any factors that are affecting you is a positive step toward improved mental and physical health.

5 Ways to Feel Happier

Easing depression can seem daunting, but there are some simple things you can do to improve your mood. That said, if your depression is severe or you are feeling suicidal, make sure to consult your doctor or therapist.

1. **Appreciate the little things.** Take note of the little things you appreciate, such as taking a long, relaxing, hot bath; lighting a candle; the smell of lavender; or going outside and gazing at the sky. Find things to be grateful for that you may have previously taken for granted, such as the happiness your pet brings you or the infinite beauty in the natural world.

2. **Help someone out.** By making others feel better, you will often help yourself feel better. This could mean leaving a simple note telling someone you work with how you value them, going above and beyond to be kind without expecting something in return, or doing the dishes when it isn't your turn. Listening and reflecting in

a meaningful way rather than venting is also often better for your mood. There can be a time and place to express displeasure, but it doesn't usually feel as productive as helping someone else.

3. **Embrace distraction.** By changing your focus, you may be able to boost your mood. For example, you might want to plan a vacation (or even just a day trip or a hike near your home), find a friend for some online Scrabble, or play a board game or cards. Joining a forum on the internet that appeals to you, such as a birding or wildflower forum, can be infinitely healthier for your mood than scrolling through political news.

4. **Find a hobby or turn to one you already have.** Check out a good book at the library, play music, try coloring or painting, take a cooking class, hone the cooking skills you already have, write in your journal, learn to build something, or learn new gardening skills. The sky's the limit for a new hobby. You might find that joining a group of people with similar hobbies is even more rewarding for your mood than going it alone.

5. **Fake it until you make it.** Smile, even if you aren't feeling like it. Laughing is even better, according to research. The simple act of moving your lips into the shape of a smile and producing a laugh can improve your mood. Walk with confidence, even if you don't feel confident. Pull your shoulders back and hold your head high. Pretend there is a string pulling your spine as straight as it can be, whether you are at your desk or walking down the street. The bonus to smiling and holding your head high is that when people see you do this, they are more likely to smile back at you, which further solidifies your feelings of happiness.

Mindfulness and Meditation

Mindfulness, or being present in the moment, brings many health benefits to your body. The most common way to practice mindfulness is through meditation. Meditation helps you clear your mind, reduce body aches and pains, and regain focus, both physically and mentally.

Here are three easy types of meditation that can be done at home or at work.

GUIDED MEDITATION

Guided meditation is a type of meditation that is done with the help of a teacher or through various apps and online videos. Each guided meditation session focuses on the mind-body-breath connection, much like yoga. Even if you are experienced at meditation, it is sometimes difficult to bring your awareness to the present without the help of a teacher.

There is a style of guided meditation for everyone, including hypnosis meditation, chakra meditation, sleep meditation, meditation for positivity, meditation to let go of negative attachments, and many more. I suggest finding a guided meditation teacher that you like, since we all respond differently to different approaches.

MINDFULNESS MEDITATION

Mindfulness meditation is simply bringing your awareness to the present using breath and relaxation. The best part about mindfulness meditation is that you can do it anywhere.

To begin, find a comfortable seat. Bring some slowness to your breath as if you were just about to fall asleep. Settle in and find as much comfort as you can without falling asleep. You may close your eyes, if you wish. Notice any mental chatter and acknowledge the thoughts and feelings that come up. While doing so, notice the sounds around you and see if these sounds can make you feel calm. Be aware of any sensations in your stomach or body and see if these sensations can make you feel calm. As you begin to feel more relaxed, try to think of a pleasant mental image of your surroundings. Think about the textures, sounds, temperatures, and images and see if these can be perceived in a whole new way.

You may be pleased to discover that you can practice a light mindfulness meditation anywhere, including while shopping, making dinner, or doing dishes. The best part about mindfulness meditation is that it doesn't require a lot of time or effort.

BODY SCAN MEDITATION

Body scan meditation is great for bringing emotional balance to the mind and body by practicing a deeper awareness of yourself. It is also used in mindfulness-based stress reduction.

You can engage in body scan meditation by sitting in a relaxed position on the floor or by lying down. I prefer a lying-down position, which helps me tune in to the different parts of my body more easily. To begin, soften your eyes or gently close them. Next, bring your awareness to your overall feelings in your body. Slow your breathing to relaxed, easy breaths through the nose. If you notice any sensations or pain in your body or mind, imagine you are bringing your breath to that area. Don't make a judgment about what you're feeling; just bring the breath to that area. Once you have brought your attention to a specific area, just observe. Then, try bringing a feeling of warmth or a color from your imagination into the area. Notice any temperature, pressure, or pulsing sensations you might be feeling and be aware of how this changes. If any emotions come up, acknowledge them and then return to the feelings your body is experiencing.

There is no right or wrong place to start scanning your body, but it's common to move from the tips of your toes all the way to the top of your head, acknowledging each part with some time and focus.

Once you have thoroughly scanned your body, take a moment to notice how your body is feeling as a whole. Continue to bring calm focus into your body for several more moments, if you can. Ideally, this whole meditation should take at least 30 minutes.

A GUT FEELING

Mental health is deeply connected to gut health. A firsthand account of this connection is shared by Lanny.

66I guess to start, I was diagnosed with bipolar schizoaffective disorder in 2011.

I dealt with a lot of depression for quite a few years, and I turned to food for comfort instead of nutrition. Alcohol and cigarettes contributed to an unhealthy lifestyle as well. My overall health declined and my weight increased.

I made the choice to cut out alcohol and cigarettes from my life about two years ago, but my unhealthy choices caught up to me and I started experiencing severe pain in my gut. It got so bad that there were many days I would just stay in bed. I had multiple visits to the doctor and a few trips to the hospital. It was a year of agony and irritation, and I was starting to feel helpless. Being in constant pain was exhausting and depressing.

I finally found hope with a new family doctor who took the time to go over nutrition, vitamins, and supplements with me. I also had success with intermittent fasting and a low-carb diet.

As my weight decreased, so did the pain in my gut. My mood increased and my energy levels started coming back. I was also having far less anxiety and depression. Now the pain that I was experiencing for about a year is gone and it has directly impacted my mental health. I rarely experience anxiety and haven't been depressed since then. I was actually discharged from seeing my psychiatrist recently, as things have been going quite well for a while.

I know now why they call the gut the second brain!99

CHAPTER 6

Putting It All Together

In this chapter, you will pull together all you have learned so far and put it into action to heal your gut. You will be following a two-week plan (or building one of your own) that incorporates healthy eating, exercise, meditation, and more.

Make sure when planning for these two weeks that you set aside time for shopping, meal preparation, and your physical and emotional health. The plan will give you ideas about how to do this, too.

Getting Started

By now, you've read a ton of information, which can seem overwhelming, but this plan will help you get started off right. Because your gut health is unique to you, you may want to adapt the plan to suit your symptoms or preferences. You know yourself best, so feel free to make adjustments as needed to ensure that you're helping your own unique microbiome in the best possible way.

The first step is to get prepared. Start this journey when you will be at home and able to prepare meals or have someone help you prepare them. Try to make sure your schedule is relatively clear of extra activities so that you can focus on self-care. Don't try to embark on this plan when you are traveling. (Eventually, though, the plan will help keep you healthy and on track when you are away from home.)

Often, stress and related gut ailments result from being run ragged and not making time to eat healthy foods, exercise, or practice meditation. You may learn that you are already taking steps to improve your health by reducing the hustle and bustle of your daily life and focusing on yourself for the next couple of weeks.

2-Week Plan

Here's the part you've been waiting for: a plan of action. By taking control of your gut health, you have the potential to heal your gut and set yourself up for good physical and mental health for the rest of your life.

A holistic approach to gut health works better than treating pieces and parts. Remember that everything in your body is connected, so you will benefit most by drawing from all areas, including eating a gut-healthy diet, doing some exercises you love, making time to get fresh air, and supplementing your diet as needed. By incorporating all aspects of self-care, you are more likely to heal faster than if you were to address only food or only exercise.

Feel free to swap meals and activities in this plan according to your preferences. For example, you can have leftovers from the previous night's meal more often than listed or switch the exercises to better fit your schedule. If you are allergic or suspect you are allergic to any of the food items in the recipes, you can find a substitute for that ingredient. In the recipes, whenever possible, I've listed alternatives to eggs and dairy, as these can be common food sensitivities. Just make sure to also adjust your shopping list to include these substitutes and alterations.

Because gluten is the most common trigger for leaky gut, all the recipes in this plan are gluten-free. While you may not ultimately have a gluten intolerance or sensitivity, it is worth trying the full elimination of gluten for three weeks or so. Even after reintroducing gluten, you may find that you simply don't miss it. That said, it may seem hard to give up your favorite bread or pasta, but keep in mind that there are great gluten-free alternatives out there.

You can repeat this plan as many times as desired. After you get used to the routine, don't hesitate to change up the particulars, but try to maintain the structure and the components: gut-healthy diet, regular exercise, meditation, and attentive self-care.

	BREAKFAST	LUNCH	DINNER
DAY 1	Vibrant Green Smoothie (page 78)	Roasted Almond and Maple-Broccoli Salad (page 108) *Make extra dressing for the salad on day 2 Herbal tea	Shrimp Enchiladas (page 124) *Make Pickled Carrots and Onions (page 97) for days 5 and 11
DAY 2	Lemon-Blueberry Muffins (page 88) Herbal tea	Carrot, Ginger, and Fennel Soup (page 113)	Leftover Shrimp Enchiladas Green salad with leftover Maple-Mustard dressing from Day 1 or vinaigrette
DAY 3	Salmon and Fennel Scramble (page 90) Herbal tea	Sauerkraut and Bell Pepper Salad (page 100)	Green Curry Beef and Vegetables (page 135)
DAY 4	Blueberry-Coconut Yogurt Bowl (page 82) Seasonal fruit Herbal tea	Lemon, Parmesan, and Kale Salad (page 107) Kombucha	Indian-Style Sprouted Lentil Curry (page 132) with rice Beet and Mint Salad (page 96)
DAY 5	Cinnamon Pancakes (page 86) *save extra batter for day 10 Kombucha	Ginger and Coriander Vegetable Beef Soup (page 116) Herbal tea	Basil Chicken Wraps with Homemade Flaxseed Tortillas (page 128) *Serve with Pickled Carrots and Onions made on day 1 Green salad
DAY 6	Lemon-Ginger Smoothie (page 79)	Leftover Ginger and Coriander Vegetable Beef Soup Herbal tea	Cod with Sauerkraut (page 123) Broccoli sprouts Sweet Potato Fries (page 104)
DAY 7	Broccoli-Cheddar Frittata (page 93) Herbal tea	Crunchy Curry Celery Salad (page 101) Herbal tea	Leftover Basil Chicken Wraps with Homemade Flaxseed Tortillas

SNACK	EXERCISE	EMOTIONAL/MENTAL HEALTH
Berry Compote (page 103) Kombucha	20-minute walk, preferably outside	Guided meditation of choice
Blueberry-Coconut Yogurt Bowl (page 82)	40 minutes of yoga	Take a bath to relax
Sweet Potato Fries (page 104)	30-minute bike ride (outside or at the gym)	Spend 20 minutes relaxing in the sun after your bike ride
Leftover Berry Compote	30 minutes of strengthening exercises	Body scan meditation to tune in to your body
Leftover Sauerkraut and Bell Pepper Salad	Rest day: stroll around the neighborhood	Dig in the dirt by gardening or tending houseplants
Yogurt Berry Salad (page 102)	30-minute hike	Double your hiking efforts by working on breathing through your nose slowly, if possible
Curry Cauliflower Pickles (page 106)	40 minutes of yoga	Mindful meditation while you do your yoga

	BREAKFAST	LUNCH	DINNER
DAY 1	Chocolate-Spinach Smoothie (page 80) Herbal tea	Stuffed Mushrooms (page 105) Kombucha	Salmon Burrito Bowls (page 121)
DAY 2	Eggs and Asparagus (page 89) Herbal tea	Lemon, Parmesan, and Kale Salad (page 107)	Ginger Shrimp Stir-Fry (page 122) with rice
DAY 3	Leftover Cinnamon Pancakes (from saved batter) Fresh fruit Herbal tea	Chicken Noodle Soup (page 115) Kombucha	Leftover Ginger Shrimp Stir-Fry
DAY 4	Sweet Potato and Poblano Hash (page 91) Herbal tea	Leftover Chicken Noodle Soup	Fermented Fried Rice with Vegetables (page 136)
DAY 5	Sunflower-Ginger Cereal (page 83) with coconut milk Herbal tea	Basil, Tomato, and Cucumber Quinoa Salad (page 110) Kombucha	Spiced Turkey Meatballs (page 138) Leftover Fermented Fried Rice with Vegetables Steamed broccoli
DAY 6	Olive Oil Breakfast Buns (page 84) Seasonal fruit Herbal tea	Eggplant and Mushroom Pizzas (page 139) Kombucha	Fresh Greens and Salmon Salad (page 98)
DAY 7	Breakfast Bake (page 92) Herbal tea	Vegetable Alfredo (page 126) Kombucha	Olive-Lemon Chicken (page 130) Green salad with maple-mustard dressing (from Roasted Almond and Maple-Broccoli Salad, page 108)

SNACK	EXERCISE	EMOTIONAL/MENTAL HEALTH
Leftover Yogurt Berry Salad	20 minutes swimming	Sit in the sun and work on slow breath work through your nose
One serving of plums or prunes	30 minutes interval training or strength training	Call a good friend or close relative
Lemon-Ginger Smoothie (page 79)	Rest day: stroll around your neighborhood	Body scan meditation
Leftover Pickled Carrots and Onions	40 minutes of yoga	Mindful meditation while you do yoga
Coconut yogurt	20 minutes brisk walking, preferably outside	Listen to some of your favorite music
Leftover Sunflower-Ginger Cereal with coconut milk	1 hour of dance or aerobics class or simply dance at home	Take time to appreciate the little things around you
Leftover Cinnamon Pancakes	30-minute hike	Dig in the dirt or care for houseplants while working on slow breathing through the nose

AFTER THE 2 WEEKS

Congratulations on completing the two-week plan! By removing common gut triggers like processed sugar and gluten, you are likely enjoying many health benefits by now. Check in with yourself. Do you have more energy? Less heartburn? Improved bowel regularity? Increased mental clarity?

I encourage you to continue the plan for an additional two weeks before reintroducing gluten. If you do find that any symptoms are amplified, pull the gluten back out of your diet, as it is likely a trigger for you. Continue to track your symptoms using the Symptom Tracker (see page 17).

You may need to make some adjustments if you aren't feeling symptom relief. A common reason for this might be that you are eating new foods and your body may need some more time to adapt. Another reason could be that you have sensitivities to other common food triggers, such as dairy, corn, or soy. You can now remove these foods or follow a full elimination diet with guidance from a registered dietitian and see how you feel during the next couple of weeks.

Troubleshooting New Symptoms

The following table is designed to help you troubleshoot any ongoing or new symptoms. Hopefully, these are minimal.

If any of your symptoms become intolerable or substantially worse, make sure to consult with your doctor. You may need to consider a more in-depth elimination diet.

Any supplements are meant to be used according to the directions for a few weeks to see if your symptoms improve. Introduce only one supplement at a time.

SYMPTOM	MODIFICATION
Diarrhea	Try cutting out dairy, corn, eggs, and soy for a week to see if your symptoms improve. Consider taking an enzyme and bile supplement combination with meals. Eat more fermented foods or take a probiotic supplement. Mix 1 teaspoon of psyllium fiber with 8 ounces of water and drink once per day. See your doctor if symptoms persist or worsen.
Light-colored stools accompanied by diarrhea or urgent stools	Try taking an enzymes and bile supplement combination with meals. See your doctor if symptoms persist.
Constipation	Drink more water. Try to eliminate dairy, corn, eggs, and soy for a week or so. Eat more fermented foods or take a probiotic supplement. Take peppermint gelcaps or drink peppermint or ginger tea. Practice breathing exercises or vagal nerve exercises like gargling or singing. Use magnesium powder daily. Consider taking a triphala supplement, which is a natural extract of three fruits used to help with constipation.
Bowel urgency	Try slowly adding more fiber, such as 1 teaspoon of psyllium, into your diet. Consider taking an enzyme and bile supplement combination with meals.
Gas	Consider removing dairy, soy, and corn for a week or so. Try cutting back on onions, chives, and garlic. Take an enzyme supplement with meals. Take a peppermint gelcap or drink a peppermint tea. Add fennel seeds to meals or teas. Chew foods slowly and thoroughly.
Bloating	Follow the tips for gas. Also, try adding more parsley, cilantro, fennel, or coriander to your dishes, as well as enzyme-rich foods like papaya and pineapple. Try an enzyme and bile supplement combination with meals.
Flatulence	Follow the tips for gas and bloating.
Burping	Chew foods more slowly and thoroughly. Eliminate dairy, corn, eggs, and soy for a week or so. Try adding apple cider vinegar to your meals or mix 1 tablespoon of apple cider vinegar with 3 tablespoons of water and drink it with meals.

SYMPTOM	MODIFICATION
Indigestion	Follow the tips for burping. Consider taking an enzyme supplement with meals.
Heartburn	Try eliminating dairy, corn, soy, and eggs for a week or so. Chew foods more slowly and thoroughly. Eat more fermented foods or take a probiotic supplement. Eliminate all caffeine. Drink a tea containing licorice root with meals for a week.
Gut pain	Drink ginger tea or eat crystallized ginger with meals. Take a peppermint gelcap or drink teas with peppermint or chamomile. Consider taking glutamine and zinc powder. N-Acetylglucosamine is an amino acid supplement that helps some people with gut pain.
Brain fog	Eliminate dairy, corn, eggs, and soy. Consider taking an all-natural multivitamin with minerals daily at mealtime.
Body aches and pains	Consider taking an all-natural multivitamin with minerals daily at mealtime. Add 1 teaspoon of chlorella powder to your smoothies. Have your doctor check your iron and vitamin D levels. Consider taking an N-Acetylglucosamine supplement. Try magnesium powder daily. Include cilantro in your diet daily.
Anxiety	Eat more fermented foods or take a probiotic supplement. Eliminate dairy, corn, eggs, and soy. Drink chamomile and herbal tea. Eliminate all caffeine. Work on slow nasal breathing and meditation.
Low energy	Have your doctor check your iron, B_{12}, and vitamin D levels. Make sure you are eating enough food. Consider taking an all-natural multivitamin with minerals daily at mealtime. Work on breathing exercises.
Food cravings or hunger	Make sure you are eating enough protein- and fiber-rich foods. Increase the portions of foods in the recommended meal plan.
Unwanted weight loss	Increase the total amount of food you are eating. Add more raw honey and healthy fats to meals. Make a bedtime smoothie. If weight loss persists, make sure to consult your doctor.

6 Tips to Stay the Course

Here are six tips to keep you on the path toward a lifetime of wellness.

1. **Build a support network.** Some people in your life may not understand what you're going through or why you're making changes in your life. Find a friend you can chat with about your gut health journey and ask them to help you stay on track. Consider reaching out to support groups in your community or a digestive health forum. By building a support network, you will have people to share successes with and who can provide encouragement when you need it.

2. **If you stray from the plan, don't beat yourself up.** Occasionally we stray from even the best of plans. Use the situation as a learning tool and withhold self-criticism or judgment. What happened that day? How did you feel? Keep track of the circumstances and your reaction in your journal. This can help you thoughtfully and intentionally overcome future challenges.

3. **Talk to your doctor and/or therapist when needed.** Health is a continuum, so there may be times when you need to seek help from your doctor, especially if you experience any sudden health changes or anything changes for the worse. Sometimes mental or physical issues may arise that are beyond your control. Seeking support from a therapist or doctor in these situations is always a good idea. It doesn't mean you have to stop following your plan; it just means that you may need some additional help or guidance.

4. **Pace yourself.** Adopting a new eating plan is best when done in a holistic way, but the reality may be that you are not ready to take on all the challenges at once. Some people experience more success with slow and gradual change. Others will do best tackling everything at once. Just remember, our microbiomes are all different, and you know yourself best. Whatever you do, don't add stress to the process by taking on too much. If you need to pace yourself, make a plan and be as consistent as you can.

5. **Listen to your body.** Paying close attention to your body's cues is more important than following any dietary or lifestyle guidelines. For example, you may be at your best after nine hours of sleep instead of seven or eight. You also may have unique sensitivities. If you know that certain foods are triggers for you, make sure to choose healthy, enjoyable alternatives. Over time, as your body heals, you can try reintroducing foods that cause sensitivities, and you may find that you tolerate them better.

6. **Use the recipes in part 3 of this book.** The recipes in this book can be part of your gut health routine from now on. These recipes are the building blocks of your new lifestyle. You will find many adaptations and tips that will help you tailor them to your specific needs. Keep in mind, these are designed to be not only healthy but also tasty!

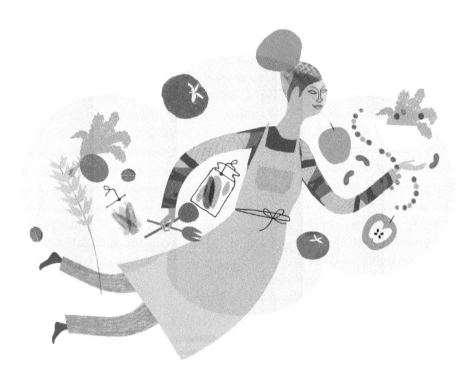

A GUT FEELING

Here is a quote from a client of mine, Julie, in regard to implementing this holistic plan for gut health:

> "I'm currently 63 years old. A combination of stressful jobs, stressful home life, and diet often left me depressed to the point of being catatonic. Honestly, there were days that the act of getting out of bed was more than I could do. I felt so sad and "heavy" and was really having difficulty finding my way forward. It all felt so hopeless sometimes. In order to function on a daily basis, I was often on and off antidepressants. Some of them worked well for me, but often the side effects were worse than the cure. I was on one so bad that coming off it was a horrific experience—one doctor called it akin to getting off heroin, and I agree. I was completely unable to concentrate or function for several weeks.
>
> It was suggested that I improve my gut health by getting off a lot of "junk." For me, this was removing refined flour of any kind and sugar from my diet and adding a couple of natural supplements and vitamins. In addition to losing weight, the change in my mental health has been remarkable. I've been on this plan for several years, and I believe my gut health has improved. It certainly has improved my overall outlook on life. I feel more energetic, more positive, and most important, I'm no longer relying on antidepressants to moderate my mood. The change has been like night and day (feels like coming out of the dark into the sunshine of the day, honestly)."

Part Three

Gut-Healing Recipes

CHAPTER 7

Breakfast and Smoothies

VIBRANT GREEN SMOOTHIE

Serves: 2   **Prep time:** 5 minutes

This smoothie tastes so refreshing, energizing, and light, you won't even know that you are getting close to 4 servings of vegetables in before noon! The celery provides gut-healing antioxidants, and some research shows it may even help regenerate nerve cells. Note that hulled hemp seeds are sometimes labeled as "hemp hearts."

2 cups unsweetened almond milk or coconut milk

2 cups kombucha or filtered water

2 tablespoons hulled hemp seeds

2 tablespoons chia seeds

6 celery stalks

4 cups fresh spinach

2 frozen bananas

1 cup fresh or frozen pineapple chunks

1 teaspoon grated fresh ginger

In a blender, combine the almond milk, kombucha, hemp seeds, chia seeds, celery, spinach, bananas, pineapple, and ginger and blend on high for about 50 seconds, or until smooth.

Tip: To make this recipe even quicker, combine all the ingredients except the banana in a sealable container the night before. Cover and refrigerate. This will also allow the chia seeds to soak, which helps your body absorb their nutrients.

Per serving: Calories: 360; Fat: 14g; Protein: 13g; Carbohydrates: 51g; Fiber: 13g; Sodium: 210mg; Iron: 5mg

LEMON-GINGER SMOOTHIE

Serves: 2   **Prep time:** 5 minutes

Lemon and ginger combine to give this smoothie an extra-fresh taste. Ginger enhances your vitamin and mineral absorption, lemon boosts the health of your intestinal lining, and hemp seeds provide you with a good amount of protein and omega-3 fatty acids.

3 cups filtered water

1⅓ cups frozen peach or mango chunks

Juice of 2 lemons

2 teaspoons grated fresh ginger

¼ cup hulled hemp seeds

2 large kale leaves, stemmed

In a blender, combine the water, peaches, lemon juice, ginger, hemp seeds, and kale and blend on high for about 30 seconds, or until smooth.

Tip: For a sweeter smoothie, add 1 teaspoon of maple syrup.

Per serving: Calories: 263; Fat: 14g; Protein: 15g; Carbohydrates: 25g; Fiber: 5g; Sodium: 15mg; Iron: 6mg

CHOCOLATE-SPINACH SMOOTHIE

Serves: 2 **Prep time:** 5 minutes

Rich in magnesium, spinach helps promote a healthy microbiome, while cocoa powder and hemp seeds are great sources of antioxidants for gut healing. If you don't love the taste of spinach, don't worry: You'll mostly taste the chocolate and peanut butter in this decadent smoothie.

2 cups coconut milk

2 tablespoons cocoa powder

2 tablespoons natural peanut butter

2 teaspoons raw honey

2 frozen bananas

6 tablespoons hulled hemp seeds

4 cups spinach

1 cucumber, cut in quarters lengthwise

2 cups ice

In a blender, combine the coconut milk, cocoa powder, peanut butter, honey, bananas, hemp seeds, spinach, cucumber, and ice and blend on high until smooth, about 30 seconds.

Tip: Add a pinch of cinnamon for an extra flavor boost.

Per serving: Calories: 560; Fat: 33g; Protein: 27g; Carbohydrates: 48g; Fiber: 10g; Sodium: 100mg; Iron: 5mg

SUNRISE LEMON-CHIA PUDDING

Serves: 2   **Prep time:** 10 minutes

This simple breakfast is bright and flavorful thanks to the lemon, honey, and berries. With this healthy dose of prebiotics and probiotics first thing in the morning, your gut will have a nourishing start to the day.

2 cups honey yogurt	Zest of 2 lemons
⅓ cup chia seeds	1 cup fresh raspberries

1. In a medium serving bowl, whisk together the yogurt, chia seeds, and lemon zest.

2. Let the pudding set for 5 to 10 minutes, then stir once more.

3. Top with the raspberries.

Tip: For a dairy-free version, use coconut milk yogurt or almond yogurt instead of traditional dairy-based yogurt. Whisk the ingredients together for an extra minute, so that the chia seeds don't clump. For a little extra natural sweetness, mix in 1 teaspoon of raw honey or maple syrup.

Per serving: Calories: 414; Fat: 15g; Protein: 19g; Carbohydrates: 56g; Fiber: 16g; Sodium: 168mg; Iron: 3mg

BLUEBERRY-COCONUT YOGURT BOWL

Serves: 2   **Prep time:** 5 minutes

This simple breakfast is so decadent that you won't even think about how healthy it is. The blueberries and avocado are rich in antioxidants and gut-friendly prebiotics to help your microbiome, while the yogurt is full of probiotics for a happy belly. The hemp seeds and peanut butter give you a good boost of protein to get you going in the morning.

2 cups plain or vanilla coconut yogurt

2 cups full-fat coconut milk

1½ cups frozen blueberries

1 avocado

2 frozen bananas

½ teaspoon cinnamon

¼ cup hulled hemp seeds

1 cup fresh or frozen raspberries

2 tablespoons natural peanut butter

1. In a blender, combine the yogurt, coconut milk, blueberries, avocado, bananas, and cinnamon and blend on high for about 30 seconds, or until smooth.

2. Put the mixture in a large bowl and top with the hemp seeds, raspberries, and peanut butter.

Tip: If you don't like the taste of coconut, try this with almond milk and almond yogurt instead.

Per serving: Calories: 435; Fat: 22g; Protein: 17g; Carbohydrates: 49g; Fiber: 9g; Sodium: 100mg; Iron: 3mg

SUNFLOWER-GINGER CEREAL

Serves: 10   **Prep time:** 5 minutes

If you are craving a crunchy, energizing cereal without all the preservatives and processed sugars, this tasty blend does the trick. Serve with your milk of choice, on its own, or enjoy as a snack.

3 cups whole-grain puffed rice

½ cup salted sunflower seeds

½ cup sprouted, salted pumpkin seeds

¼ cup chia seeds

¼ cup raw honey

¼ cup natural peanut butter

½ teaspoon ground ginger

¼ teaspoon nutmeg

1. In a large mixing bowl, combine the puffed rice, sunflower seeds, pumpkin seeds, and chia seeds.
2. In a small bowl, mix together the honey, peanut butter, ginger, and nutmeg.
3. Add the honey mixture to the puffed rice and seeds and stir well to coat.
4. Store leftovers in an airtight container in the refrigerator for up to 1 month.

Tip: If you need to avoid peanut butter, substitute almond or sunflower butter.

Per serving: Calories: 158; Fat: 10g; Protein: 5g; Carbohydrates: 15g; Fiber: 3g; Sodium: 80mg; Iron: 2mg

OLIVE OIL BREAKFAST BUNS

Makes: 12 buns   **Prep time:** 15 minutes, plus 2 hours to rise   **Cook time:** 20 minutes

I love a savory breakfast bun, but they are usually made with gluten, which can be rough on your gut. You can mix this dough together the day before and keep it in your refrigerator until you are ready to bake.

2 cups all-purpose gluten-free flour

¼ cup chia seeds

¼ cup coconut flour

1 tablespoon yeast

4 tablespoons extra-virgin olive oil, divided, plus more for greasing

¼ or ½ teaspoon Himalayan pink salt

5 large eggs, at room temperature

½ cup warm water

1½ tablespoons apple cider vinegar

½ cup kalamata olives, sliced (optional)

1 or 2 tablespoons balsamic vinegar (optional)

1 tablespoon Italian seasoning

1. In a large mixing bowl or using a stand mixer, combine the all-purpose flour, chia seeds, coconut flour, yeast, 2 tablespoons of olive oil, salt (use only ¼ teaspoon if you are using olives), eggs, water, apple cider vinegar, and olives (if using).

2. Mix until the dough is stiff, yet somewhat sticky. If the dough is too sticky, add a bit more flour. Cover the dough and allow it to rise at room temperature for about 1 hour.

3. Preheat the oven to 350°F. Grease a 12-cup muffin tin with olive oil.

4. Scoop out 2 heaping tablespoons of dough and shape them into a single ball. Place the ball into a muffin cup. (The dough should be peeking up slightly over the top of the tin.) Repeat with the remaining dough. Loosely cover the muffin tin with plastic wrap. Once again, allow the dough to rise for about 1 hour.

5. Bake the buns for about 20 minutes, or until tops are slightly golden.

6. Meanwhile, in a small bowl, whisk together the remaining 2 tablespoons of olive oil, the balsamic vinegar (if using), and Italian seasoning. Serve the warm buns with the Italian vinaigrette for dipping.

Per serving (2 buns): Calories: 270; Fat: 6g; Protein: 13g; Carbohydrates: 35g; Fiber: 9g; Sodium: 380mg; Iron: 2mg

CINNAMON PANCAKES

Makes: 8 pancakes   **Prep time:** 15 minutes   **Cook time:** 10 minutes

This recipe, adapted from The Paleo Running Mama website, provides all the indulgent flavors and richness of your favorite cinnamon rolls, minus the unwanted sugar spikes and crashes. This version is low in sugar and high in protein and includes antioxidant-rich cinnamon and nutmeg.

FOR THE PANCAKES
5 large eggs, room temperature

⅓ cup full-fat coconut milk

3 tablespoons melted ghee or coconut oil, plus more for greasing the griddle

1 tablespoon freshly squeezed lemon juice or apple cider vinegar

3 tablespoons maple syrup

1 teaspoon vanilla extract

⅓ cup coconut flour

½ cup arrowroot flour or all-purpose gluten-free flour

¾ teaspoon baking soda

¼ teaspoon salt

1½ teaspoons cinnamon

FOR THE CINNAMON SYRUP
⅔ cup full-fat coconut milk

⅓ cup maple syrup

1 tablespoon cinnamon

⅛ teaspoon nutmeg

TO MAKE THE PANCAKES

1. Preheat a griddle or cast-iron skillet over medium heat.

2. In a large mixing bowl, whisk together the eggs, coconut milk, ghee, lemon juice, maple syrup, and vanilla.

3. Stir in the coconut flour, arrowroot flour, baking soda, and salt, making sure to mix well so that there are no clumps of baking soda in the mix.

4. Gently fold in the cinnamon to make cinnamon streaks throughout the batter. (Do not mix vigorously.) The batter should be moderately thick, but not so thick that it can't be poured. If needed, thin with a little extra coconut milk.

5. Pour a little melted coconut oil into the pan, then pour about ⅓ cup batter onto the heated griddle.

6. Cook each pancake for 4 to 5 minutes on each side, or until the pancake is cooked through.

TO MAKE THE CINNAMON SYRUP

7. While the pancakes are cooking, in a small saucepan, whisk together the coconut milk, maple syrup, cinnamon, and nutmeg.

8. Bring the syrup mixture to a boil, then reduce the heat to low. Simmer for 3 to 5 minutes, or until the syrup reaches your desired consistency.

9. When the pancakes are done, transfer them to a serving plate and drizzle the hot cinnamon syrup over the top.

Tip: This recipe tastes even better if you make the batter ahead and refrigerate it for 2 to 3 days before cooking. This will allow some fermentation to begin. You can keep the batter covered in the refrigerator for up to 1 week and bring it out anytime you want a pancake.

Per serving (2 pancakes): Calories: 362; Fat: 22g; Protein: 8g; Carbohydrates: 35g; Fiber: 3g; Sodium: 308mg; Iron: 2mg

LEMON-BLUEBERRY MUFFINS

Makes: 12 muffins **Prep time:** 10 minutes **Cook time:** 20 minutes

Muffins are often just as sugary and full of processed ingredients as cake, but this gut-friendly version uses anti-inflammatory olive oil, extra eggs for gut-repairing protein, maple syrup for 24 different types of antioxidants, and a mix of coconut and whole-grain gluten-free flour for microbiome-friendly fiber and fats. Replace the olive oil with coconut oil or ghee if you prefer. You can also use honey instead of maple syrup.

⅔ cup extra-virgin olive oil, plus more for greasing

½ cup coconut flour

½ cup all-purpose whole-grain gluten-free flour

¼ teaspoon salt

½ teaspoon baking powder

5 large eggs, at room temperature

5 ounces plain coconut yogurt

⅓ cup maple syrup

Juice of 1 lemon

Zest of 1 lemon (optional)

¾ cup blueberries

1. Preheat the oven to 350°F. Grease a 12-cup muffin tin lightly with olive oil.

2. In a large mixing bowl, combine the coconut flour, all-purpose flour, salt, and baking powder and mix thoroughly.

3. Add the eggs, olive oil, yogurt, maple syrup, lemon juice, and lemon zest (if using). Mix until thoroughly combined.

4. Fold in the blueberries.

5. Evenly distribute the batter into the muffin cups.

6. Bake for 15 to 18 minutes, or until the top of the muffin is springy yet soft.

Tip: For an egg-free version, substitute 1¼ cups of carbonated water for the eggs.

Per serving (2 muffins): Calories: 419; Fat: 30g; Protein: 8g; Carbohydrates: 31g; Fiber: 5g; Sodium: 219mg; Iron: 2mg

EGGS AND ASPARAGUS

Serves: 4   **Prep time:** 5 minutes   **Cook time:** 10 minutes

Broiling the asparagus really brings out its flavor in this easy-to-make dish that can be enjoyed for any meal of the day. Asparagus is rich in prebiotic fibers and contains at least 100 beneficial compounds, including antioxidants. Serve with Olive Oil Breakfast Buns (page 84) or whole-grain gluten-free toast.

1 pound asparagus, cut into 2-inch pieces

2 teaspoons extra-virgin olive oil

4 large eggs

Pinch salt

1. Put an oven rack in the middle position. Set the oven to broil.
2. Arrange the asparagus pieces in the bottom of an 8-by-8-inch baking dish. Drizzle with the olive oil and toss well to coat.
3. Broil the asparagus on high for 4 to 5 minutes, or until tender. Remove the dish from the oven.
4. Crack the eggs, one at a time, over the asparagus mixture, allowing a small amount of space between each egg.
5. Put the dish back into the oven and broil for 3 to 4 minutes more for a slightly runny yolk or 5 minutes for a firm yolk.
6. Remove from the oven and season with the salt.

Tip: Keep a close eye on the eggs: They can look undercooked even when they are not because they develop a shine when cooking.

Per serving: Calories: 192; Fat: 13g; Protein: 14g; Carbohydrates: 6g; Fiber: 3g; Sodium: 128mg; Iron: 4mg

SALMON AND FENNEL SCRAMBLE

Serves: 4   **Prep time:** 5 minutes   **Cook time:** 10 minutes

Start your day off right with this salmon dish packed with protein and omega-3s. Caraway and fennel impart flavor and provide antioxidants that can reduce symptoms of irritable bowel syndrome.

1 tablespoon butter or ghee

1 cup chopped fennel bulb

½ teaspoon whole caraway seeds

6 large eggs

2 tablespoons half-and-half

4 ounces wild smoked salmon

¼ teaspoon salt

Freshly ground black pepper

2 tablespoons minced chives, for garnish

2 tablespoons minced fennel fronds, for garnish

1. In a medium skillet, melt the butter over medium heat. Add the chopped fennel bulb and caraway seeds and cook for 5 to 6 minutes, or until the fennel bulb has softened.

2. Meanwhile, in a medium mixing bowl, whisk together the eggs and half-and-half.

3. Flake the salmon into bite-size pieces.

4. Transfer the cooked fennel to a plate and set aside.

5. Put the skillet back on the stove over medium-high heat. Pour in the eggs, stirring continuously, so the mixture doesn't stick. Scramble the eggs for 1 to 2 minutes, or until they are fluffy.

6. Reduce the heat to low and add the fennel mixture back to the pan, along with the smoked salmon. Stir the mixture together to combine, just until all ingredients are warmed through.

7. Turn the heat off. Season with the salt and a grind or two of pepper. Sprinkle the chives and the fennel fronds over the scramble to garnish.

Per serving: Calories: 147, Fat: 9g, Protein: 14g, Carbohydrates: 3g, Fiber: 1g; Sodium: 480mg; Iron: 1mg

SWEET POTATO AND POBLANO HASH

Serves: 4   **Prep time:** 5 minutes   **Cook time:** 15 minutes

This hash makes a quick but satisfying meal that you can eat anytime of day. The combination of antioxidant-rich vegetables, sweet potatoes, and spices helps reduce inflammation, and the aged cheese provides a probiotic source for your microbiome. Substitute Italian seasoning and fennel for the coriander and Southwest seasoning or bell pepper for poblanos, if you want to vary the flavors.

2 tablespoons extra-virgin olive oil

2 medium sweet potatoes, diced

½ large sweet onion, diced

2 large poblano chiles, seeded and diced

¼ teaspoon salt

1 teaspoon coriander seeds

2 teaspoons Southwest seasoning

1 cup shredded sharp cheddar cheese

1. In a large skillet, heat the olive oil over medium heat.

2. Add the sweet potatoes, onion, and poblanos and season with the salt.

3. Add the coriander and Southwest seasoning and mix well.

4. Put a lid over the pan and cook for 10 to 12 minutes, stirring occasionally.

5. Once the sweet potatoes have softened, remove the lid, and top the mixture with the cheese.

Tip: For a dairy-free version with even more protein, leave out the cheese, lightly beat 3 large eggs, then scramble them into the hash during the last couple of minutes of cooking.

Per serving: Calories: 285; Fat: 17g; Protein: 9g; Carbohydrates: 26g; Fiber: 4g; Sodium: 368mg; Iron: 1mg

BREAKFAST BAKE

Serves: 6   **Prep time:** 5 minutes   **Cook time:** 30 minutes

Hearty breakfast bakes like this can deliver a ton of nutrition. Free-range eggs pack in vitamins, while all-natural sausage adds protein and zinc for gut healing.

1 tablespoon extra-virgin olive oil

½ pound fresh spinach

¼ teaspoon salt

1 cup diced tomatoes (about 2 medium)

½ pound all-natural breakfast sausage

½ large onion, diced

1 teaspoon dried rosemary

1 teaspoon fennel seeds

1½ cups diced zucchini (about 2 small)

8 large eggs

1. Preheat the oven to 350°F. In a large oven-safe skillet, preferably cast iron, heat the olive oil over medium-high heat.

2. Add the spinach and sauté for 1 to 2 minutes, or until the leaves wilt and turn bright, shiny green.

3. Put a colander in the sink. Transfer the spinach to the colander and allow the moisture to drain off.

4. Salt the tomatoes, then add them to the colander to drain.

5. Using the same skillet over medium heat, cook the sausage, onion, rosemary, and fennel seeds for about 8 minutes.

6. Squeeze any water out of the spinach and tomato mixture.

7. Add the zucchini, tomatoes, and spinach to the pan and mix thoroughly. Heat until warm, about 2 minutes.

8. Whisk the eggs together, then pour them over the vegetable and sausage mixture.

9. Transfer the skillet to the oven and bake for about 20 minutes, or until the eggs are set and cooked through.

Per serving: Calories: 240; Fat: 18g; Protein: 15g; Carbohydrates: 5g; Fiber: 2g; Sodium: 750mg; Iron: 3mg

BROCCOLI-CHEDDAR FRITTATA

Serves: 6　**Prep time:** 10 minutes　**Cook time:** 15 minutes

A weekend favorite, this frittata is light, puffy, and satisfyingly cheesy. It's also packed with probiotics and antioxidants.

1 tablespoon extra-virgin olive oil

8 large eggs

½ teaspoon salt

½ teaspoon freshly ground black pepper

½ cup cultured buttermilk

½ teaspoon dried mustard powder

1 sweet onion, chopped

3 cups broccoli florets, thinly sliced

1 large garlic clove, minced

1 cup grated sharp cheddar cheese

1 tablespoon chopped fresh herbs or 1 teaspoon dried herbs

1 bag broccoli sprouts or broccoli sprout mix

1. Preheat the oven to 425°. In a large cast-iron or ceramic skillet, heat the olive oil over medium heat.

2. While the oil is heating, whisk together the eggs, salt, pepper, buttermilk, and dried mustard powder.

3. Add the onion to the skillet and sauté for 3 to 4 minutes, or until slightly translucent.

4. Add the broccoli and garlic to the skillet and sauté for another 1 to 2 minutes. Turn off the heat.

5. Pour the egg mixture over the vegetables. (Do not stir.) Top with the cheese and herbs.

6. Put the skillet in the oven and bake for 10 to 12 minutes, or until the eggs are firm yet springy. Remove the frittata from the oven and let it sit for about 5 minutes.

7. Using a pizza cutter, slice the frittata into 8 wedges. Serve each slice with 2 tablespoons of broccoli sprouts.

Per serving: Calories: 197; Fat: 13g; Protein: 14g; Carbohydrates: 7g; Fiber: 2g; Sodium: 431mg; Iron: 2mg

CHAPTER 8

Soups, Salads, and Sides

BEET AND MINT SALAD

Serves: 2   **Prep time:** 8 minutes

Raw beets and fresh mint are a great way to get more color into your diet while providing lots of antioxidants for your gut. The mint in this recipe may help reduce gas pain and bloating. Serve this salad with aged cheese or walnuts (or both) to make it into a light meal or serve it as a side with Cod with Sauerkraut (page 123).

4 medium beets (about 1 pound)	2 tablespoons fresh mint, chopped	2 tablespoons apple cider vinegar
½ cup diced red onion	2 teaspoons brown mustard	2 tablespoons extra-virgin olive oil

1. Peel the beets.

2. Using a grater, grate the beets onto a cutting board or plate.

3. Put the beets, onion, and mint into a large serving bowl.

4. In a small bowl, whisk together the mustard, vinegar, and olive oil.

5. Pour the mustard vinaigrette over the top of the beet mixture and toss well to coat the vegetables.

Tip: If you dislike mint, feel free to use tarragon or basil instead.

Per serving: Calories: 214; Fat: 14g; Protein: 3g; Carbohydrates: 19g; Fiber: 5g; Sodium: 130mg; Iron: 1mg

PICKLED CARROTS AND ONIONS

Serves: 8   **Prep time:** 10 minutes, plus 30 minutes to cool   **Cook time:** 5 minutes

Homemade pickled vegetables are quick to make, and they taste better than most store-bought pickles while having less salt. The unfiltered apple cider vinegar in this recipe includes the mother, which provides additional probiotic benefits, while the vegetables give your gut prebiotics. These pickles taste best after a day or two in the refrigerator, so make a batch ahead of time and keep them at the ready to serve with recipes like Basil Chicken Wraps with Home-made Flaxseed Tortillas (page 128) or for a quick snack.

1½ cups apple cider vinegar, with the mother

1½ cups water

1 teaspoon salt

2 large garlic cloves, crushed

3 bay leaves

½ teaspoon whole peppercorns

½ teaspoon dill seed

¼ teaspoon celery seed

1 pound whole carrots, peeled and cut into matchsticks

½ red onion, cut into ⅛-inch-thick slices

1. In a small saucepan over high heat, combine the vinegar, water, and salt. Bring to a boil, then remove from the heat.

2. In a quart jar, such as a canning jar, add the garlic, bay leaves, peppercorns, dill, and celery seed. Add the carrots and onion to the jar, alternating so that they are in layers. You will need to push them all down, but they all should fit into the jar tightly.

3. Pour the hot vinegar mixture into the jar over the vegetables. The liquid should cover the vegetables.

4. Allow the liquid to cool in the jar for about 30 minutes.

5. Seal the jar and store in the refrigerator for up to 2 months.

Tip: Vary the herb mixture by adding coriander, cumin, or oregano (but always include bay leaves, because they help keep the vegetables crisp).

Per serving: Calories: 35; Fat: 1g; Protein: 1g; Carbohydrates: 6g; Fiber: 2g; Sodium: 186mg; Iron: 1mg

FRESH GREENS AND SALMON SALAD

Serves: 2   Prep time: 10 minutes   Cook time: 5 minutes

This light and crisp salad is citrusy, savory, and satisfying. Even my children, who are often skeptical of fish, love this recipe. Many store-bought salad dressings contain hidden inflammatory ingredients, such as soybean or canola oil, but this recipe uses a simple, delicious mix of olive oil and lemon juice.

2 (4-ounce) salmon fillets

2 tablespoons extra-virgin olive oil, divided

¾ cup finely diced sweet onion, divided

¼ teaspoon paprika

½ teaspoon dill weed

Pinch salt (optional)

6 cups mixed greens

1 cup chopped kale or cabbage

3 tablespoons freshly squeezed lemon juice, divided

1 teaspoon gluten-free Worcestershire sauce

Freshly ground black pepper (optional)

Lemon wedges, for serving

1. Using paper towels, pat the salmon dry.

2. In a large skillet, heat 1 teaspoon of olive oil over medium-high heat. Add ½ cup of onion and sauté for 5 to 7 minutes, or until the onion begins to brown.

3. Place the fillets on top of the onions.

4. Brush the top of each fillet with 2 teaspoons of oil and season them with paprika, dill, and salt (if using).

5. After about 3 minutes, or when the pan side of the fish is opaque, turn the fillets over.

6. While the fish is cooking, put the mixed greens and kale into a large bowl.

7. Sprinkle the remaining ¼ cup of onion over the salad and dress the greens with the remaining 1 teaspoon of olive oil and 2 tablespoons of lemon juice.

8. Splash the fillets with the Worcestershire sauce and the remaining 1 tablespoon of lemon juice.

9. Cover the pan and reduce the heat to low for 2 minutes, or until the fish flakes easily with a fork.

10. Flake the fillets into bite-size pieces.

11. Put the flaked salmon and cooked onions on top of the lettuce mixture. Season with salt and pepper, if using. Serve with lemon wedges.

Tip: Feel free to add other vegetables to the salad, such as chopped fresh tomatoes, cucumbers, or anything else you enjoy and have on hand.

Per serving: Calories: 343; Fat: 22g; Protein: 25g; Carbohydrates: 13g; Fiber: 4g; Sodium: 227mg; Iron: 2mg

SAUERKRAUT AND BELL PEPPER SALAD

Serves: 6   **Prep time:** 5 minutes

While sauerkraut and bell pepper might seem like an odd pairing, their sweet and sour flavors are a delicious combination. Your microbiome will get a big boost thanks to the sauerkraut's probiotics and the bell pepper's prebiotics. Store, covered, in the refrigerator for up to 1 week. Serve it alongside a gluten-free sandwich for lunch or as a side to a hearty main dish of chicken, fish, or meat.

2 cups raw sauerkraut

1 red bell pepper, chopped

½ sweet onion, chopped

2 tablespoons extra-virgin olive oil

2 tablespoons maple syrup

Juice of 1 lemon

In a medium mixing bowl, combine the sauerkraut, bell pepper, onion, olive oil, maple syrup, and lemon juice and mix thoroughly.

Tip: You can find raw sauerkraut in the refrigerator section of grocery stores. Make sure to buy the kinds without preservatives.

Per serving: Calories: 80; Fat: 5g; Protein: 1g; Carbohydrates: 10g; Fiber: 2g; Sodium: 210mg; Iron: 1mg

CRUNCHY CURRY CELERY SALAD

Serves: 2   Prep time: 15 minutes

Celery is an unsung hero when it comes to health. It has a high anti-oxidant content, it may reduce chances of getting stomach ulcers, and it may even help improve nerve health. The cherries, curry powder, black pepper, dill, and onion in this extra-crunchy salad also provide gut-healing antioxidants. Serve this as a lunch entrée or mix in some roasted chicken to make it a more robust meal.

2 cups finely sliced celery

½ cup thinly sliced red onion

¼ cup salted roasted almonds

¼ cup dried cherries

1 teaspoon curry powder

⅓ cup avocado mayonnaise

½ teaspoon freshly ground black pepper

4 cup chopped leafy greens

Fresh dill, minced, for garnish (optional)

1. In a medium mixing bowl, mix together the celery, onions, almonds, and cherries.

2. In a small bowl, combine the curry powder, mayonnaise, and pepper. Mix until well combined.

3. Spoon the curry dressing over the vegetables and toss until all the vegetables are coated.

4. Serve the curried celery salad over the greens.

5. Garnish with fresh dill, if using.

Tip: If you are allergic to eggs, you can mix together 3 tablespoons of mashed avocado and 3 tablespoons of olive oil and substitute it for the mayonnaise.

Per serving: Calories: 295; Fat: 18g; Protein: 8g; Carbohydrates: 30g; Fiber: 8g; Sodium: 378mg; Iron: 2mg

YOGURT BERRY SALAD

Serves: 4 **Prep time:** 10 minutes

This fruit salad combines fresh fruits with a creamy dressing for a satisfying side or dessert. It's full of healthy gut-healing antioxidants thanks to the mint, cinnamon, lemon juice, and a rainbow of apples, grapes, berries, and cherries. Do not substitute Greek yogurt—you will need a thinner-textured yogurt for the mixture to coat the fruit evenly.

⅔ cup nondairy yogurt, honey or plain

½ teaspoon cinnamon

Juice of 1 lemon

1 tablespoon maple syrup

1 Granny Smith apple, diced

1 cup red grapes

1 cup blueberries

¼ cup dried cherries

1 tablespoon fresh mint, finely chopped (optional)

1. In a medium mixing bowl, mix together the yogurt, cinnamon, lemon juice, and maple syrup.

2. Add the apple, grapes, blueberries, and cherries. Fold the mixture together until the fruit is coated in the yogurt dressing.

3. Sprinkle with the mint, if using.

Tip: You can use regular yogurt in this recipe if you tolerate dairy.

Per serving: Calories: 143; Fat: 1g; Protein: 2g; Carbohydrates: 33g; Fiber: 3g; Sodium: 30mg; Iron: 1mg

BERRY COMPOTE

Serves: 4   **Prep time:** 5 minutes   **Cook time:** 10 minutes

On your journey to good gut health, you can still enjoy something sweet during the day without suffering from the adverse effects of traditional sugary snacks. This berry treat keeps your gut health on track by providing antioxidants and prebiotics. While it tastes great on its own, you can also pour it over yogurt or try it on gluten-free pancakes.

2 cups berries of your choice   **¼ cup real maple syrup**   **Juice of 1 lemon**

1. In a medium saucepan, combine the berries, maple syrup, and lemon juice.
2. Over medium heat, bring the compote to a boil, stirring occasionally.
3. Reduce the heat to low and simmer for 5 minutes, or until the liquid has slightly reduced and the compote has thickened.
4. Remove from the heat and enjoy.

Tip: You can use plums or peaches for this recipe instead of the berries or any combination of these fruits.

Per serving: Calories: 105; Fat: 1g; Protein: 1g; Carbohydrates: 27g; Fiber: 3g; Sodium: 3mg; Iron: 1mg

SWEET POTATO FRIES

Serves: 2 **Prep time:** 10 minutes **Cook time:** 20 minutes

This recipe will satisfy your fried food cravings without the harmful fats. These fries are packed with gut-healing anti-inflammatory compounds from both the sweet potatoes and the olive oil.

3 tablespoons extra-virgin olive oil

1 large sweet potato

¼ cup all-purpose gluten-free flour

1½ teaspoons garlic powder, divided

2 teaspoons dried oregano, divided

3 tablespoons avocado mayonnaise

Zest of 1 lemon

1. Preheat the oven to 425°F. Line a baking sheet with aluminum foil. Pour the olive oil onto the foil and spread it out evenly.

2. Leaving the skin on, cut the sweet potato into ¼-by-¼-inch fries.

3. In a medium mixing bowl, mix together the flour, 1 teaspoon of garlic powder, and 1 teaspoon of oregano.

4. Dredge each sweet potato fry in the flour mixture.

5. Place each sweet potato fry onto the prepared sheet pan, then roll it over in the oil, thoroughly coating the breading. Make sure that you leave plenty of space between the fries so they will bake evenly.

6. Bake for 10 minutes. Meanwhile, in a small bowl, make the aioli by whisking together the mayonnaise, lemon zest, remaining 1 teaspoon of oregano, and remaining ½ teaspoon of garlic powder.

7. Remove the fries from the oven and flip them over, making sure they remain separated. Put the fries back in the oven and bake for an additional 8 to 10 minutes, or until they are browned.

8. Season with salt, if desired. Allow the fries to rest for about 5 minutes. Serve with the aioli for dipping.

Per serving: Calories: 273; Fat: 16g; Protein: 3g; Carbohydrates: 29g; Fiber: 4g; Sodium: 160mg; Iron: 1mg

STUFFED MUSHROOMS

Serves: 4   Prep time: 10 minutes   Cook time: 25 minutes

These stuffed mushrooms make a great appetizer or light lunch served with a salad. Mushrooms are great for digestive health because they are rich in minerals like selenium and zinc and they provide prebiotics. Meanwhile, the filling uses goat cheese, which is easier to digest than cheese made from cow's milk.

8 large button mushrooms

4 ounces chèvre goat cheese, softened

3 tablespoons olive oil, divided

2 garlic cloves, minced

⅛ teaspoon cayenne pepper (optional)

⅛ teaspoon paprika

¼ cup sweet onion, finely chopped

1. Preheat the oven to 425°F.

2. Remove the stems from the mushrooms and finely chop them.

3. In a small mixing bowl, combine the goat cheese, 2 tablespoons of olive oil, garlic, cayenne (if using), and paprika. Set aside.

4. In a medium skillet, heat the olive oil over medium heat. Add the onion and chopped mushroom stems. Sauté for about 5 minutes, or until the onions are lightly browned.

5. Remove the vegetables from the heat and stir them into the cheese mixture.

6. Spoon the cheese and vegetable filling into the mushroom caps. (You can heap the mixture above the caps.)

7. Place the mushrooms onto a baking sheet and bake for about 20 minutes, or until the mushrooms are bubbly and lightly browned on top.

Tip: Experiment with adding some lemon zest, which goes well with the flavor of the goat cheese, or add some Parmesan for an extra flavor boost.

Per serving: Calories: 180; Fat: 17g; Protein: 7g; Carbohydrates: 2g; Fiber: 1g; Sodium: 107mg; Iron: 1mg

CURRY CAULIFLOWER PICKLES

Serves: 8   **Prep time:** 5 minutes, plus 30 minutes to cool   **Cook time:** 5 minutes

Cauliflower stays crisper in the refrigerator when pickled than cucumbers and is just as tasty as a snack, side, or salad topping. With the addition of curry powder and extra spices, these cauliflower pickles reduce inflammation in your gut and throughout your whole body. These taste best if you allow them to sit in the refrigerator for 3 to 4 days before eating them.

1 cup apple cider vinegar, with the mother

1 cup filtered water

2 teaspoons non-iodized salt

2 teaspoons curry powder

½ teaspoon mustard powder

1 tablespoon extra-virgin olive oil

2 large garlic cloves, crushed

2 bay leaves

2 teaspoons coriander seeds

1 small head cauliflower, cut into 1- to 2-inch pieces

1. In a medium saucepan over high heat, combine the vinegar, water, salt, curry powder, mustard powder, and olive oil. Bring the mixture to a boil, then remove from the heat.

2. In a quart jar, such as a canning jar, add the garlic, bay leaves, and coriander seeds.

3. Add all the cauliflower to the jar, pushing the florets down tightly so that they all fit.

4. Pour the hot vinegar mixture into the jar over the cauliflower. The liquid should cover all the florets.

5. Allow the liquid to cool in the jar for about 30 minutes.

6. Seal the jar and store in the refrigerator for up to 1 month.

Tip: You can reduce the salt, if you wish, but be aware that the cauliflower won't keep as long.

Per serving: Calories: 31; Fat: 2g; Protein: 1g; Carbohydrates: 4g; Fiber: 1g; Sodium: 150mg; Iron: 1mg

LEMON, PARMESAN, AND KALE SALAD

Serves: 4 **Prep time:** 8 minutes, plus 20 minutes to rest

Rich in the antioxidant sulforaphane, kale is a superfood for gut health, and it becomes more bioavailable when combined with the mustard. With a little probiotic from the yogurt and lots of prebiotics from the honey and vegetables, this salad is a great way to nourish your microbiome.

½ cup freshly squeezed lemon juice

Zest of 1 lemon

½ cup extra-virgin olive oil

¼ cup honey yogurt

2 teaspoons raw honey

2 teaspoons Dijon or brown mustard

¼ teaspoon salt

½ cucumber, diced

½ cup shredded Parmesan cheese

6 cups chopped red kale

1. In a blender, combine the lemon juice, lemon zest, olive oil, yogurt, honey, mustard, and salt. Blend until smooth and creamy, about 30 seconds.

2. In a large mixing bowl, combine the cucumber, Parmesan, and kale, then spoon about half the lemon dressing over it.

3. Allow the salad to sit for 15 to 20 minutes so that the flavors can absorb into the kale.

4. Store any extra dressing in a sealed bottle in the refrigerator for up to 1 week and use as a sauce or on other salads.

Tip: Use nondairy yogurt and omit the cheese if you are allergic or sensitive to dairy.

Per serving: Calories: 340; Fat: 31g; Protein: 7g; Carbohydrates: 11g; Fiber: 1g; Sodium: 398mg; Iron: 1mg

ROASTED ALMOND AND MAPLE-BROCCOLI SALAD

Serves: 6   **Prep time:** 10 minutes, plus overnight for the almonds to soak
Cook time: 2 hours 45 minutes

This crunchy and gut-healthy salad goes the extra mile: By soaking and slow-roasting the raw almonds, the anti-nutrients and toxins are removed from the almonds to make them easier to digest and their nutrients become easier to absorb. As the nuts soak, they swell up a bit, and the water will turn brownish. This is how you know that the soaking process is working.

FOR THE ALMONDS
3 tablespoons Himalayan pink salt or sea salt

3 cups filtered water

1 pound raw almonds

FOR THE SALAD
5 cups chopped broccoli

½ cup chopped sweet onion

¼ cup raisins or dried cranberries

3 tablespoons extra-virgin olive oil

2 tablespoons apple cider vinegar

2 tablespoons maple syrup

1 tablespoon Dijon mustard

¼ teaspoon salt

½ teaspoon freshly ground black pepper

TO MAKE THE ALMONDS

1. In a medium mixing bowl, combine the salt and the filtered water. Mix well. Add the almonds, cover, and let rest on the counter overnight.

2. Preheat the oven to 170°F. Line a baking sheet with parchment paper.

3. Drain the almonds and put them on the prepared baking sheet. Put them in the oven and allow them to dehydrate for about 2 hours.

4. Increase the heat to 250°F and roast for another 45 minutes.

5. Remove from the oven and allow to cool. Chop ½ cup of almonds for the salad and store the rest in a sealed bag in a cupboard for up to 1 month.

TO MAKE THE SALAD

6. In a medium mixing bowl, combine the chopped almonds, broccoli, onion, and raisins.

7. In a small bowl, whisk together the olive oil, vinegar, maple syrup, mustard, salt, and pepper.

8. Pour the dressing over the salad and toss to coat.

Tip: For a salad with fewer carbs, reduce the maple syrup to 1 tablespoon and omit the dried fruit.

Per serving: Calories: 197; Fat: 13g; Protein: 5g; Carbohydrates: 18g; Fiber: 4g; Sodium: 249mg; Iron: 1mg

BASIL, TOMATO, AND CUCUMBER QUINOA SALAD

Serves: 6 **Prep time:** 8 minutes, plus 8 to 12 hours for the quinoa to ferment
Cook time: 15 minutes

Quinoa has some anti-nutrients and can be bitter, but a great solution to this is to ferment it. By soaking it in water and vinegar, the bitter compounds are removed while also improving the available nutrients for absorption. The fennel, basil, and mint in this recipe will help temper IBS symptoms, too. Try this with Cod with Sauerkraut (page 123) or serve chilled for a light, refreshing lunch.

FOR THE QUINOA
1½ cups red quinoa

1 tablespoon apple cider vinegar with the mother

FOR THE SALAD
2¾ cups water

1 teaspoon salt, divided

1½ teaspoons fennel seeds, crushed

1 heaping tablespoon minced garlic, minced

4 tablespoons extra-virgin olive oil

1 tablespoon brown or Dijon mustard

1 teaspoon freshly ground black pepper

2 tablespoons apple cider vinegar with the mother

1 cucumber, diced

1 medium tomato, diced

2 tablespoons basil, minced

1½ teaspoons fresh mint, minced

TO FERMENT THE QUINOA

1. Using a colander, rinse the quinoa.

2. Transfer the quinoa to a medium glass mixing bowl and cover it with filtered water. Mix in 1 tablespoon of apple cider vinegar and allow to ferment for about 8 to 12 hours, or overnight.

3. Using a colander, drain and rinse the quinoa.

TO MAKE THE SALAD

4. In a medium saucepan over high heat, combine the drained quinoa, the water, ½ teaspoon of salt, the fennel seeds, and the garlic. Bring the liquid to a boil, skimming off and discarding any foam that may develop.

5. Reduce the heat to low and simmer for about 15 minutes, or until all the water is absorbed.

6. Meanwhile, in a small mixing bowl, mix together the olive oil, mustard, pepper, remaining ½ teaspoon of salt, and vinegar.

7. Transfer the cooked quinoa to a medium mixing bowl. Allow it to cool for about 5 minutes, then pour the dressing over it and mix well.

8. Stir in the cucumber, tomato, basil, and mint.

9. Serve warm or refrigerate for about 1 hour before serving for a chilled salad.

Tip: Try varying the herbs by using combinations like tarragon and thyme instead of the basil and mint.

Per serving: Calories: 252; Fat: 12g; Protein: 7g; Carbohydrates: 30g; Fiber: 4g; Sodium: 421mg; Iron: 2mg

SAUTÉED BRUSSELS SPROUTS AND HERBS

Serves: 5   **Prep time:** 5 minutes   **Cook time:** 10 minutes

This recipe has become a household favorite. Rich in sulforaphane, the antioxidant that is also found in broccoli sprouts, Brussels sprouts help reduce inflammation in the gut and the whole body. Try serving this with Spiced Turkey Meatballs (page 138), but it pairs well with any main dish and even makes a great appetizer. Leave out the cheese if you are allergic or sensitive to dairy.

1 tablespoon extra-virgin olive oil

1 pound Brussels sprouts, sliced thin

1 teaspoon Italian seasoning

¼ teaspoon dried mustard

Pinch salt

3 tablespoons Parmesan cheese

1. In a large skillet, heat the olive oil over medium heat. Add the Brussels sprouts, Italian seasoning, dried mustard, and salt.

2. Sauté for 6 to 7 minutes, stirring occasionally. The sprouts should begin to soften and the thinner pieces will begin to get crispy.

3. Top with the Parmesan cheese and continue to cook for 1 to 2 minutes, or until the Brussels sprouts reach your desired crispness.

Tip: Vary the spice mixture by trying dried thyme and sage, lemon, or a Southwest seasoning blend instead of the Italian seasoning.

Per serving: Calories: 80; Fat: 4g; Protein: 4g; Carbohydrates: 10g; Fiber: 4g; Sodium: 38mg; Iron: 2mg

CARROT, GINGER, AND FENNEL SOUP

Serves: 4   Prep time: 5 minutes   Cook time: 20 minutes

This tasty and nourishing soup is a simple lunch to make on a weekend. The fennel and caraway help alleviate gut pain and symptoms of IBS. Carrots, onions, and broccoli sprouts are rich in antioxidants that reduce gut inflammation, too. Double the batch if you'd like to have leftovers for lunches during the week.

2 tablespoons extra-virgin olive oil	2 cups sliced carrots	½ teaspoon salt
½ sweet onion, diced	1 tablespoon minced garlic	⅓ cup cultured sour cream
1½ teaspoons fennel seeds	1 teaspoon grated fresh ginger	Broccoli sprouts, for garnish (optional)
½ teaspoon caraway seeds (optional)	3 cups chicken bone broth	

1. In a medium saucepan, heat the olive oil over medium heat. Add the onion, fennel seeds, caraway seeds (if using), and carrots and cook for about 5 minutes, or until the onion begins to turn translucent.

2. Stir in the garlic and ginger and cook for another 1 to 2 minutes, or until the garlic is fragrant.

3. Add the broth and salt and increase the heat to high. Bring the liquid to a boil.

4. Reduce the heat to low and simmer for about 10 minutes, or until the carrots have softened.

5. Remove from the heat and stir in the sour cream.

6. Carefully transfer the soup to a blender. Puree the soup until smooth, about 20 seconds.

7. Top with a handful of broccoli sprouts, if using.

Tip: Use nondairy sour cream substitute if you are allergic or sensitive to dairy.

Per serving: Calories: 156; Fat: 11g; Protein: 8g; Carbohydrates: 9g; Fiber: 2g; Sodium: 418mg; Iron: 1mg

HOT AND SOUR MUSHROOM VEGETABLE SOUP

Serves: 4 **Prep time:** 5 minutes **Cook time:** 10 minutes

Mushrooms are a superstar food for gut health because they deliver prebiotics, vitamins, antioxidants, and minerals. Find beech mushrooms, if possible, because they contribute wonderful flavor and texture to this soup; otherwise, button mushrooms are a good choice. To make this soup a bit spicier, dice up a jalapeño and add it with the Anaheim chile in step 2.

1 (8-ounce) package beech mushrooms or button mushrooms

2 tablespoons extra-virgin olive oil

1 large sweet onion, chopped

1 large Anaheim chile, julienned

1 large carrot, julienned

3 cups chicken bone broth

¼ cup apple cider vinegar, with the mother

½ teaspoon salt

⅓ cup cultured sour cream

1. In a large saucepan over medium heat, combine the mushrooms, olive oil, and onion and sauté for 5 to 6 minutes, or until the onions become translucent and the mushrooms are tender.
2. Add the chile and carrot. Continue to sauté for another 2 minutes.
3. Stir in the broth, vinegar, and salt. Increase the heat to high heat and bring the soup to a boil.
4. Reduce the heat to low and simmer for another 1 to 2 minutes, or until the carrots are crisp-tender.
5. Turn off the heat and stir in the sour cream.

Tip: Omit the sour cream or use nondairy sour cream if you are allergic or sensitive to dairy.

Per serving: Calories: 165; Fat: 11g; Protein: 9g; Carbohydrates: 8g; Fiber: 2g; Sodium: 389mg; Iron: 1mg

CHICKEN NOODLE SOUP

Serves: 8   Prep time: 5 minutes   Cook time: 35 minutes

This chicken noodle soup is gut-friendly thanks to bone broth, which is a natural source of protein, glutamine, collagen, and minerals like magnesium, calcium, and zinc.

4 large celery stalks, cut into ½-inch-thick slices

1 sweet onion, chopped

1 pound (around 4 medium) carrots, cut into ½-inch-thick slices

2 tablespoons extra-virgin olive oil

1½ teaspoons dried rosemary, crushed

½ teaspoon dried sage or 1 teaspoon fresh sage, minced

3 large garlic cloves, minced

2 teaspoons Himalayan pink salt

2 bay leaves

1½ pounds boneless, skinless chicken breasts, cut into bite-size pieces

8 cups chicken bone broth

2 cups gluten-free noodles

Zest and juice of 1 lemon

Salt

Freshly ground black pepper

1. In a large saucepan, combine the celery, onion, carrots, olive oil, rosemary, and sage over medium-low heat. Cover and sweat the vegetables, stirring occasionally, for about 8 minutes. Add the garlic and salt, then re-cover the pan and cook for about 2 minutes more, or until the vegetables are fork-tender.

2. Increase the heat to high and add the bay leaves, chicken, and broth. Bring the liquid to a boil uncovered. Once it begins to boil, reduce the heat to low and simmer for 10 minutes.

3. Mix in the gluten-free noodles and cook for another 10 to 12 minutes, or until the noodles are al dente.

4. Add the lemon juice and lemon zest. Remove the bay leaves, and season with salt and pepper to taste.

Per serving: Calories: 250; Fat: 6g; Protein: 29g; Carbohydrates: 19g; Fiber: 5g; Sodium: 830mg; Iron: 1mg

GINGER AND CORIANDER VEGETABLE BEEF SOUP

Serves: 6   Prep time: 8 minutes   Cook time: 20 minutes

A twist on classic vegetable beef soup, this recipe tastes great on a fall or winter evening. By using grass-finished beef and bone broth, this soup gives you a boost of antioxidants, gut-healing proteins, and glutamine. A blend of healthy vegetables and garlic also helps support the immune system. Curry Cauliflower Pickles (page 106) are a nice complement to the flavors of this dish.

1½ pounds grass-finished ground beef

½ large onion, chopped

2 large carrots, sliced

1 tablespoon coriander seeds, crushed

1 tablespoon minced garlic

1 teaspoon grated fresh ginger

2 poblano chiles, diced

1 (15-ounce) can tomato sauce

3 cups beef bone broth

1 cup water

½ teaspoon salt

1 bunch fresh cilantro, chopped

1. In a large saucepan over medium heat, brown the ground beef.

2. Add the onion, carrots, and coriander seeds and sauté for another 5 minutes, or until the onions have softened.

3. Add the garlic and ginger and sauté for another minute.

4. Mix in the poblanos, tomato sauce, broth, water, and salt. Increase the heat to high and bring the soup to a boil.

5. Reduce the heat to low and simmer for about 15 minutes, or until the carrots have softened.

6. Ladle into serving bowls and sprinkle each generously with fresh cilantro.

Tip: Make this soup ahead and simmer on a warming unit until ready to serve.

Per serving: Calories: 356; Fat: 23g; Protein: 26g; Carbohydrates: 12g; Fiber: 4g; Sodium: 540mg; Iron: 4mg

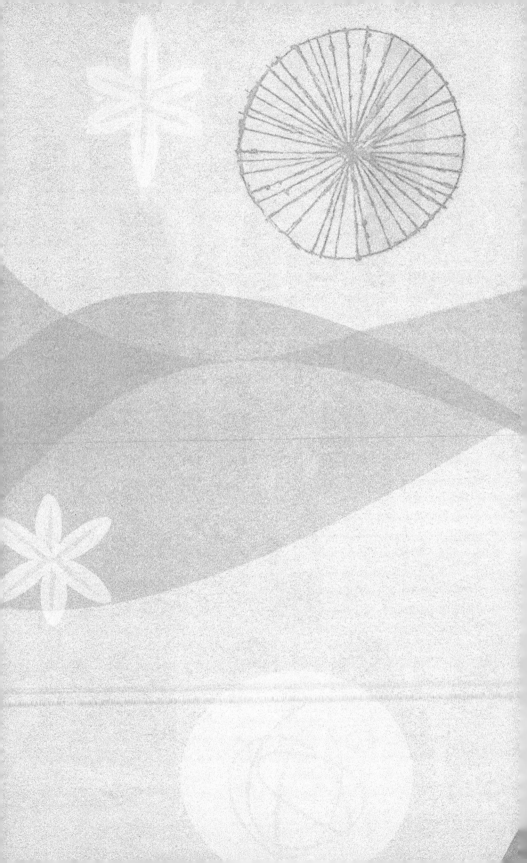

CHAPTER 9

Main Dishes

MEDITERRANEAN SALMON

Serves: 4   **Prep time:** 5 minutes   **Cook time:** 25 minutes

An easy yet elegant dinner, this salmon recipe is full of omega-3s that help reduce the risk of inflammatory bowel diseases and support a healthy microbiome for immune function.

4 (4-ounce) salmon fillets, about 1 inch thick

Pinch salt

2 tablespoons extra-virgin olive oil

2 large tomatoes, diced

1 tablespoon minced garlic

Zest of 1 lemon

¼ cup kalamata olives

Freshly ground black pepper

1. Preheat the oven to 400°F. Line a baking sheet with parchment paper.

2. Place the salmon fillets together, skin-side down, on half of the prepared baking sheet. Season the fillets with the salt, then fold the parchment over and wrap the fillets in the paper, tucking the edges underneath the fillets.

3. Bake the fillets for 15 to 25 minutes, or until the salmon flakes easily with a fork.

4. Meanwhile, in a medium saucepan, heat the olive oil over medium heat. Add the tomatoes, garlic, lemon zest, and olives.

5. Bring to a low boil and simmer for 3 to 5 minutes, or until the sauce is heated through. Season with salt and pepper.

6. Reduce the heat to low to keep the sauce warm until the fish is done cooking.

7. Place each fillet on a plate, topping each with about ½ cup of the sauce.

8. Season with a little more freshly ground black pepper, if desired.

Per serving: Calories: 255; Fat: 16g; Protein: 24g; Carbohydrates: 5g; Fiber: 1g; Sodium: 380mg; Iron; 1mg

SALMON BURRITO BOWLS

Serves: 4   **Prep time:** 15 minutes   **Cook time:** 10 minutes

Burrito bowls are healthier versions of burritos because they don't have the processed grains of the traditional wraps. To make this even healthier, use fermented rice, following the cooking method in the recipe for Fermented Fried Rice with Vegetables (page 136).

2 jalapeños, seeded

2 bunches cilantro, coarsely chopped, plus more for garnish

½ cup cultured sour cream

Juice of 2 limes

1 teaspoon dried oregano

½ cup extra-virgin olive oil, plus 1 tablespoon

Salt

Freshly ground black pepper

4 (4-ounce) salmon fillets

1½ teaspoons Southwest seasoning

1 teaspoon coriander seeds

2 cups cooked rice

8 cups chopped romaine lettuce

1 large heirloom tomato, diced

1 (15-ounce) can organic corn, drained

1. In a blender, combine the jalapeños, cilantro, sour cream, lime juice, oregano, and ½ cup of olive oil and blend until smooth, about 45 seconds. Season with salt and pepper. Set aside.

2. In large skillet, heat the remaining 1 tablespoon of oil over medium heat. Place the fillets in the pan. Season the fillets with the Southwest seasoning, coriander seeds, salt, and pepper.

3. Cook for about 3 minutes on each side, or until the fish flakes easily with a fork.

4. Place ½ cup of rice, 2 cups of lettuce, ¼ cup of the tomato, a quarter of the corn, and 1 salmon fillet in each bowl.

5. Top with cilantro sauce and garnish with a few leaves of cilantro.

Tip: To reduce the carbohydrates, simply omit the rice, which brings this down to 32g per bowl.

Per serving: Calories: 640; Fat: 29g; Protein: 32g; Carbohydrates: 45g; Fiber: 6g; Sodium: 100mg; Iron: 3mg

GINGER SHRIMP STIR-FRY

Serves: 4 **Prep time:** 10 minutes **Cook time:** 10 minutes

Ginger gives this recipe a little kick and benefits the gut by increasing digestive motility and the absorption of nutrients. The vegetables provide prebiotics, while the shrimp provides protein and omega-3s for gut healing and immunity. To complete the meal, serve this dish with fermented rice (page 136).

¼ cup tamari or coconut aminos

½ cup chicken bone broth

1 teaspoon sesame oil

2 teaspoons grated fresh ginger, divided

4 garlic cloves, grated, divided

2 tablespoons extra-virgin olive oil, divided

4 cups broccoli florets

2 cups thinly sliced carrots

1 sweet onion, sliced

½ pound shrimp, shelled and deveined

⅛ teaspoon red pepper flakes (optional)

1. In a small mixing bowl, whisk together the tamari, broth, sesame oil, 1 teaspoon of ginger, and half of the garlic. Set aside.

2. In a large skillet or wok, heat 1 tablespoon of olive oil over medium-high heat. Add the broccoli, carrots, and onion, and sauté, stirring constantly, for 2 to 3 minutes, or until the vegetables are crisp-tender.

3. Transfer the vegetables to a large bowl.

4. Return the skillet to the heat and pour in the remaining 1 tablespoon of olive oil. Add the shrimp and the remaining half of the garlic and 1 teaspoon of ginger, as well as the red pepper flakes (if using). Cook the shrimp for 1 to 2 minutes, or until pink on one side. Flip the shrimp and cook for an additional 1 to 2 minutes, or until opaque.

5. Put the vegetables back into the skillet and pour in the tamari sauce. Cook for about 2 minutes, or until the vegetables and sauce are heated through.

Per serving: Calories: 228; Fat: 9g; Protein: 15g; Carbohydrates: 24g; Fiber: 5g; Sodium: 513mg; Iron: 2mg

COD WITH SAUERKRAUT

Serves: 4   **Prep time:** 5 minutes   **Cook time:** 15 minutes

Cod is a very lean fish that is rich in the antioxidant selenium, which is critical for immune function in the gut and for bringing down inflammation. Probiotic and antioxidant ingredients in this recipe will give your gut a boost.

2 tablespoons olive oil, divided

½ sweet onion, diced

1 cup raw sauerkraut

2 tablespoons capers

⅓ cup chicken bone broth

½ teaspoon dill seed

4 (4-ounce) wild cod fillets

Pinch salt

2 tablespoons all-purpose gluten-free flour

½ cup cultured sour cream

2 tablespoons chives, minced, for garnish

1. In a small saucepan, heat 1 tablespoon of olive oil over medium heat. Add the onion and sauté for about 5 minutes, or until the onion has softened.

2. Stir in the sauerkraut, capers, bone broth, and dill seed and bring the broth to a boil. Reduce the heat to low and simmer for about 10 minutes.

3. Meanwhile, in a cast-iron skillet, heat the remaining 1 tablespoon of olive oil over medium heat.

4. Pat the cod fillets dry with a paper towel, then season them with salt. Coat each fillet in flour.

5. Place the fillets into the skillet and cook for about 5 minutes on each side, or until the fish flakes easily with a fork.

6. Add the sour cream to the sauerkraut mixture and mix well. Heat until warm. Turn off the heat.

7. Place each fillet on a serving plate topped with the sauerkraut mixture, and garnish with chives.

Per serving: Calories: 240; Fat: 14g; Protein: 22g; Carbohydrates: 5g; Fiber: 1g; Sodium: 482mg; Iron: 1mg

SHRIMP ENCHILADAS

Serves: 6   **Prep time:** 15 minutes   **Cook time:** 40 minutes

With lots of spices and extra-virgin olive oil, these enchiladas are full of flavor and rich in antioxidants that help reduce inflammation in the gut. Bone broth and shrimp provide gut-healing minerals like zinc and selenium that also contribute to the reduction of inflammation, along with glutamine, which nourishes the gut lining.

3 tablespoons all-purpose gluten-free flour

4 tablespoons extra-virgin olive oil, divided

3 tablespoons Southwest seasoning, divided

2 cups chicken bone broth

Salt

Freshly ground black pepper

1 large jalapeño, seeded and minced

1 (15-ounce) can sweet corn

¾ cup diced sweet onion

1 pound small shrimp, shelled and deveined

½ cup cultured sour cream

12 corn tortillas

1. In a small saucepan over medium heat, whisk together the flour, 3 tablespoons of olive oil, and 2 tablespoons of Southwest seasoning. Cook for about 2 minutes, whisking constantly, until bubbly and aromatic.

2. Whisk in the chicken broth and bring to a boil.

3. Reduce the heat to low and simmer for 3 to 4 minutes, or until the sauce has thickened.

4. Add a pinch of salt and pepper.

5. Move the sauce to a warming unit to keep warm until you are ready to pour it over the enchiladas.

6. Preheat the oven to 350°F.

7. In a large skillet, heat the remaining 1 tablespoon of oil over medium heat. Add the jalapeño, corn, and onion. Sauté for 5 minutes, or until the onion has softened and is translucent.

8. Add the shrimp, then stir in the remaining 1 tablespoon of Southwest seasoning.

9. Sauté for 2 to 3 minutes, or until the shrimp turn pink and are cooked through.
10. Turn off the heat and stir in the sour cream.
11. In a small skillet, heat the corn tortillas over medium heat until softened, about 40 seconds each.
12. Place about ¼ cup of the shrimp mixture in the center of each tortilla. Gently roll up each tortilla and place it, seam-side down, in a 10-by-13-inch baking dish.
13. Once all of the filled tortillas are nestled in the dish, pour the enchilada sauce over the top.
14. Bake for 30 minutes.

Tip: Use dairy-free sour cream if you are allergic or sensitive to dairy.

Per serving: Calories: 394; Fat: 17g; Protein: 24g; Carbohydrates: 40g; Fiber: 5g; Sodium: 755mg; Iron: 3mg

VEGETABLE ALFREDO

Serves: 4   Prep time: 10 minutes   Cook time: 15 minutes

This version of Alfredo can be made in less than 30 minutes, and it won't feel like a gut bomb. It provides microbiome-supporting prebiotics from the shiitakes, vegetables, garlic, and lemon. The zucchini replaces traditional pasta in this dish, but feel free to serve it over cooked whole-grain rice pasta, if desired.

¾ cup heavy (whipping) cream

2 large garlic cloves, minced, divided

1¼ cups grated Parmesan cheese

2 tablespoons extra-virgin olive oil

2 cups sliced shiitake mushrooms

1 red bell pepper, diced

2 medium large zucchini, peeled lengthwise in ribbons

1 teaspoon grated lemon zest

¼ teaspoon salt

¼ teaspoon freshly ground black pepper

2 tablespoons chives, minced, for garnish

2 tablespoons parsley, chopped, for garnish

1. In a small saucepan, heat the cream and half of the garlic over medium-low heat.

2. Stir in the Parmesan cheese. Once the cheese has melted, reduce the heat to low and keep warm until ready to use.

3. Heat a large skillet over medium heat. Pour in the olive oil, then add the mushrooms and stir. Sauté the mushrooms for about 5 minutes, or until softened.

4. Add the bell pepper and the remaining garlic. Cook for another 1 to 2 minutes, or until the garlic is fragrant.

5. Add the zucchini ribbons, lemon zest, salt, and pepper. Cook for 1 to 2 minutes, or until heated through.

6. Place one-quarter of the vegetables on each serving plate.

7. Top with 2 to 3 tablespoons of Alfredo sauce and garnish with the chives and parsley.

Tip: For dairy-free Alfredo sauce, in a small saucepan, whisk together 1 teaspoon of cornstarch and 1 cup of full-fat coconut milk. Stir in ½ cup of chicken stock and simmer until thickened.

Per serving: Calories: 403; Fat: 33g; Protein: 16g; Carbohydrates: 15g; Fiber: 4g; Sodium: 680mg; Iron: 1mg

BASIL CHICKEN WRAPS WITH HOMEMADE FLAXSEED TORTILLAS

Serves: 8   **Prep time:** 30 minutes, plus 2 to 4 hours for the flaxseed to ferment
Cook time: 30 minutes

Using fermented flaxseed may sound odd at first, but they make the texture and flavor of these tortillas perfect, not to mention they're full of healthy omega-3s and prebiotic fibers to reduce inflammation and support a healthy microbiome. Avocados, onion, and basil increase the health of the gut lining. If you made a jar of Pickled Carrots and Onions (page 97) in advance, add them to this dish to make the flavors pop.

FOR THE TORTILLAS
⅔ cup flaxseed meal

⅔ cup filtered water, plus ½ cup

1 teaspoon apple cider vinegar, with the mother

2 cups all-purpose gluten-free flour, plus more for dusting

½ teaspoon salt

2 tablespoons coconut oil, melted

1 tablespoon extra-virgin olive oil, plus more for frying

FOR THE WRAPS
1 tablespoon extra-virgin olive oil

1½ pounds boneless, skinless chicken breasts

Salt

Freshly ground black pepper

½ sweet onion, sliced

1 tablespoon minced garlic

1 ripe avocado, mashed with a pinch of salt

1 large tomato, diced

4 cups chopped lettuce

2 tablespoons basil leaves, stemmed

1 cup Pickled Carrots and Onions (page 97, optional)

TO MAKE THE TORTILLAS

1. In a small mixing bowl, mix together the flaxseed meal, ⅔ cup of filtered water, and vinegar. Allow the flaxseed to ferment at room temperature for 2 to 4 hours.

2. In a large mixing bowl, mix together the gluten-free flour, ½ cup of filtered water, salt, coconut oil, and the fermented flaxseed. When the dough begins to get stiff, knead it until all of the ingredients are fully incorporated. If the dough is not stiff, add a little extra flour, as needed.

3. Dust a clean, flat surface with gluten-free flour to prevent the dough from sticking. Roll a piece of dough into a 2-inch ball and put it on the floured work surface.

4. Using a rolling pin, roll out the dough until it is about 10 inches in diameter. Sprinkle with more flour as needed to prevent the dough from sticking to the rolling pin.

5. In a large skillet, heat the olive oil over medium heat. Place the tortilla in the pan and cook for 2 minutes. Flip the tortilla and cook for another minute.

6. Repeat until the tortillas are all cooked, adding more olive oil as needed to prevent sticking.

7. Cover the tortillas with a clean kitchen towel and set them aside until you are ready to make the wraps.

TO MAKE THE WRAPS

8. In a large skillet, heat the olive oil over medium heat. Add the chicken and season with a pinch of salt and pepper.

9. Cook the chicken for about 2 minutes on each side, or until lightly browned and cooked through.

10. Add the onion and garlic. Cook for another 2 to 4 minutes, or until the onions have begun to soften.

11. Spread about 1 tablespoon of the avocado down the center of a tortilla. Top with ¼ cup of chicken, 2 tablespoons of tomatoes, ½ cup of lettuce, 1 teaspoon of basil, and ½ cup of pickled carrots and onion (if using).

12. Roll the wraps snugly in a tube shape about 2 inches in diameter.

13. Cut each wrap in half to serve.

Tip: If you are pressed for time, substitute store-bought gluten-free tortillas for the homemade flaxseed tortillas.

Per serving: Calories: 402; Fat: 20g; Protein: 25g; Carbohydrates: 30g; Fiber: 10g; Sodium: 250mg; Iron: 3mg

OLIVE-LEMON CHICKEN

Serves: 6   Prep time: 15 minutes   Cook time: 4 to 6 hours

In this recipe, slow cooking mellows the olives while giving the chicken an extra-rich flavor. Coriander and fennel seeds historically have been used to help reduce bloating and other digestive ailments, and research supports their use for these purposes.

2 tablespoons extra-virgin olive oil, divided

2 pounds boneless, skinless chicken breasts

1 teaspoon fennel seeds

2 teaspoons coriander seeds

Juice of 3 lemons

1 cup pitted olives, a mix of both green and kalamata

1 cup beech mushrooms or button mushrooms

1½ cups chicken bone broth

1. In a large skillet, heat 1 tablespoon of olive oil over medium heat. Add half of the chicken.

2. Cook the chicken for about 3 minutes on each side, or until just browned. Transfer the chicken to a plate. Repeat with the remaining chicken.

3. Put the chicken in a slow cooker with the fennel and coriander seeds, lemon juice, olives, mushrooms, and remaining 1 tablespoon of olive oil. Pour in the broth.

4. Cook on low for 4 to 6 hours.

Tip: To make this in an Instant Pot, at step 4, set the Instant Pot to Pressure Cook and cook for 25 minutes.

Per serving: Calories: 269; Fat: 12g; Protein: 34g; Carbohydrates: 7g; Fiber: 2g; Sodium: 643mg; Iron: 1mg

COCONUT CHICKEN

Serves: 4   **Prep time:** 5 minutes   **Cook time:** 50 minutes

This dish is inspired by a recipe my mom makes, but I made some simple adaptations to boost its gut benefits. Coconut milk contains medium-chain triglycerides, a great type of fat for the gut. Bone-in chicken thighs have more gut-healing nutrients than chicken breasts and more collagen that supports gut healing.

½ tablespoon ghee or extra-virgin olive oil

1 sweet onion, sliced

1 garlic clove, minced

4 bone-in chicken thighs (remove the skin, if desired)

½ tablespoon dried oregano

¼ teaspoon dried sage

1 teaspoon salt

½ teaspoon freshly ground black pepper

2 cups full-fat coconut milk

½ cup chicken bone broth

1. In a large cast-iron skillet, warm the ghee over medium heat. Add the onion and garlic and sauté for about 3 minutes, or until the onion has just begun to soften.

2. Add the chicken and brown for about 6 minutes, then flip the thighs and cook for about 6 minutes more.

3. Season the chicken with oregano, sage, salt, and pepper.

4. Pour in the coconut milk and bone broth. As you are bringing the liquid to a low boil, scrape up the brown bits from the bottom of the pan.

5. Reduce the heat to low and simmer for 35 minutes, or until the chicken and vegetables are tender. Check the pan every 10 minutes or so to make sure the mixture isn't sticking to the skillet.

6. Taste and adjust the seasoning, if needed.

Per serving: Calories: 343; Fat: 27g; Protein: 17g; Carbohydrates: 8g; Fiber: 1g; Sodium: 378mg; Iron: 3mg

INDIAN-STYLE SPROUTED LENTIL CURRY

Serves: 8   **Prep time:** 15 minutes, plus 24 hours for the lentils to sprout
Cook time: 25 minutes

Sprouted lentils are much tastier and healthier than unsprouted lentils, because the sprouting process removes anti-nutrients, allows for better nutrient absorption, and reduces gas and bloating. It also speeds up the cooking time of the lentils. At a minimum, make sure to soak the lentils and any other legumes you consume for a couple hours to reduce the anti-nutrients they contain. Sprouted lentils require less soaking time than many other sprouted foods.

FOR THE SPROUTED LENTILS
1 pound dried lentils

FOR THE CURRY
4 tablespoons butter or ghee

½ large red onion, chopped

1 tablespoon coriander seeds

1 cup carrots, cut into ½-inch slices

1 cup fresh green beans, cut into 1-inch slices

1 cup frozen or fresh corn

1 teaspoon turmeric (optional)

1 tablespoon curry powder

3 tablespoons tomato paste

2 large garlic cloves, minced

1 teaspoon ground cardamom

1 teaspoon salt

3 cups water

TO SPROUT THE LENTILS

1. Put the lentils into a large saucepan. Cover them with two inches of water and allow them to soak for 2 to 4 hours.

2. Drain the lentils and return them to the pan. Cover the pan and let the lentils sit for about a day.

3. After a day has passed, a small sprout should be emerging from each lentil.

4. Rinse and drain the lentils. Return them to the pan again and cover them with 2 inches of water.

5. Bring the water to a boil over high heat and cook for about 5 minutes, or until the lentils have softened.

TO MAKE THE CURRY

6. In a separate large saucepan, melt the butter over medium heat. Add the onion and coriander seeds and sauté for about 5 minutes, or until the onion has softened.

7. Mix in the carrots, green beans, and corn. Sauté for another 2 to 4 minutes, or until the beans have slightly softened.

8. Add the turmeric (if using). Then, mix in the curry powder, tomato paste, and garlic. Cook for another 1 to 2 minutes, or until fragrant.

9. Add the cardamom and salt along with 4 cups of the cooked, sprouted lentils and the water and bring everything to a boil.

10. Reduce the heat to low, cover, and simmer for 5 to 10 minutes, or until the lentils have absorbed most of the water but the curry is still slightly liquid.

11. Freeze any extra lentils in a freezer-safe container for up to 6 months.

Tip: Use other vegetables in this recipe, if desired, such as kale, spinach, sweet potatoes, or fresh tomatoes.

Per serving: Calories: 192; Fat: 5g; Protein: 10g; Carbohydrates: 28g; Fiber: 10g; Sodium: 309mg; Iron: 4mg

BEEF AND VEGETABLE STEW

Serves: 5   **Prep time:** 15 minutes   **Cook time:** 1 hour 15 minutes

In this gut-healing version of classic American beef stew, apple cider vinegar doubles as a fermented food and a meat tenderizer. Substitute all-purpose gluten-free flour for the cornstarch if you are allergic or sensitive to corn. Serve with a side of mashed potatoes or fermented rice (page 136) and a green salad to complete the meal.

1 tablespoon extra-virgin olive oil	3 thyme sprigs or ½ teaspoon dried thyme	¼ head cabbage, cut into roughly 2-inch pieces
1½ pounds grass-finished beef stew meat	2 rosemary sprigs or 1 teaspoon dried rosemary	2 or 3 large kale leaves, ribs removed, chopped
½ cup apple cider vinegar, with the mother	4 carrots, peeled and cut into 1-inch pieces	1 tablespoon cornstarch
1½ cups beef bone broth or mushroom broth	4 celery stalks, cut into 1-inch pieces	¼ cup water Salt
1 onion, quartered		Freshly ground black pepper

1. In a large skillet or Dutch oven, heat the olive oil over medium heat. Add the beef and cook for 2 to 3 minutes on each side, or until browned.

2. Stir in the apple cider vinegar, broth, onion, thyme, and rosemary. Cover and reduce the heat to low. Simmer for about 45 minutes.

3. Add the carrots and celery, replace the lid, and cook for another 20 minutes.

4. Add the cabbage and kale, replace the lid once more, and cook for an additional 10 minutes.

5. In a small bowl, whisk together the cornstarch and water, add the mixture to the pan, and stir until the liquid has thickened, about 1 minute. Season with salt and pepper.

Per serving: Calories: 279; Fat: 10g; Protein: 34g; Carbohydrates: 12g; Fiber: 3g; Sodium: 400mg; Iron: 4mg

GREEN CURRY BEEF AND VEGETABLES

Serves: 4   **Prep time:** 10 minutes   **Cook time:** 15 minutes

This green curry provides a huge variety of antioxidants that help improve gut immunity. Feel free to use chicken or fish in this versatile recipe, too; just make sure to reduce the cooking time for fish. Serve with fermented rice (page 136), if desired.

1 pound grass-finished sirloin steak, thinly sliced

½ large onion, sliced

1½ cups sliced button mushrooms

1 (15-ounce) can full-fat coconut milk

½ cup water

1 to 2 tablespoons green curry paste

1 to 2 tablespoons raw honey

3 cups broccoli florets

1 red bell pepper, sliced

Pinch salt

1. In a large saucepan over medium-high heat, combine the steak, onion, mushrooms, coconut milk, water, green curry paste, and honey and bring to a boil.
2. Reduce the heat to low, cover, and simmer for 10 minutes.
3. Add the broccoli and bell pepper, return the lid to the pan, and continue to simmer for 5 minutes, or until the broccoli is fork-tender.
4. Season with salt.

Tip: The green curry paste is spicy, so reduce the amount of curry paste for a milder sauce.

Per serving: Calories: 319; Fat: 13g; Protein: 28g; Carbohydrates: 21g; Fiber: 3g; Sodium: 171mg; Iron: 3mg

FERMENTED FRIED RICE WITH VEGETABLES

Serves: 10 **Prep time:** 10 minutes, plus 12 to 24 hours for the rice to ferment
Cook time: 45 minutes

One of the easiest foods to ferment is rice, and its fermentation is a great way to get some extra probiotics. The fermentation also makes the rice better for the gut lining. If you plan ahead, making fermented rice is a breeze. Simply set it on the counter the night before you plan to make this dish (or any other using fermented rice). If you're unable to ferment the rice, you can make regular brown rice. This dish makes extra and is great as leftovers the next day, or it can be served as a side with dishes like Green Curry Beef and Vegetables (page 135).

FOR THE FERMENTED RICE
2 cups brown rice

7 cups of filtered water, divided

1 teaspoon distiller's or baker's yeast (optional)

FOR THE FRIED RICE
2 tablespoons extra-virgin olive oil

1 cup chopped carrots

1 sweet onion, chopped

1 poblano chile, diced

1 cup chopped kale, chopped

1 tablespoon minced garlic

4 large eggs

3 tablespoons tamari

2 tablespoons sesame oil

TO MAKE THE FERMENTED RICE

1. Put the rice in a large mixing bowl. Add 4 cups of filtered water to cover and allow the rice to sit for 12 to 24 hours. Add the yeast, if using, to speed up the fermentation process.

2. Drain the rice.

3. In a medium saucepan, combine the rice and remaining 3 cups of filtered water. Bring to a boil over high heat.

4. Cover the pan, reduce the heat to low, and simmer for 30 to 35 minutes.

TO MAKE THE FRIED RICE

5. In a large skillet, heat the olive oil over medium heat. Add the carrots and onion and sauté for about 5 minutes, or until tender.

6. Mix in the poblano, kale, and garlic. Sauté for another 2 minutes.

7. Increase the heat to medium-high and add the eggs, stirring continuously. Cook for about 2 minutes, or until most of the moisture from the eggs has been absorbed.

8. Turn off the heat and mix in the tamari and the sesame oil.

Tip: Mix in some roasted chicken or tempeh for some extra protein, if desired.

Per serving: Calories: 384; Fat: 11g; Protein: 9g; Carbohydrates: 62g; Fiber: 6g; Sodium: 427mg; Iron: 2mg

SPICED TURKEY MEATBALLS

Serves: 4   **Prep time:** 5 minutes   **Cook time:** 20 minutes

Resembling a Swedish meatball but with extra spice and zest to kick up the flavors, these are a light dinner full of gut-healthy ginger, lemon, and cardamom. Research shows that cardamom helps with nausea and may even reduce your risk of developing stomach ulcers.

1 pound ground turkey

⅓ cup grated Parmesan cheese

1 teaspoon ground cardamom

1 teaspoon ground ginger

¼ cup gluten-free rolled oats

2 tablespoons chives, minced

¼ teaspoon salt

½ teaspoon freshly ground black pepper

Zest of 1 lemon

1 large egg

1 tablespoon butter or ghee

1 tablespoon all-purpose gluten-free flour

1 cup chicken bone broth

Salt

Freshly ground black pepper

1. Preheat the oven to 350°F. Line a baking sheet with aluminum foil.

2. In a large mixing bowl, combine the turkey, Parmesan, cardamom, ginger, oats, chives, salt, pepper, lemon zest, and egg. Mix well.

3. Shape the meat mixture into 1½- to 2-inch balls, then place them on the prepared baking sheet so that they are evenly spaced.

4. Bake for 15 to 18 minutes, or until browned.

5. Meanwhile, in a small saucepan, melt the butter over medium heat. Whisk in the flour and cook for about 1 minute, or until the mixture is bubbling.

6. Whisk in the chicken broth and cook the gravy for 3 to 5 minutes, or until it reaches a low boil. Season with salt and pepper. Serve the meatballs smothered in gravy.

Per serving: Calories: 211; Fat: 6g; Protein: 34g; Carbohydrates: 5g; Fiber: 1g; Sodium: 379mg; Iron: 1mg

EGGPLANT AND MUSHROOM PIZZAS

Serves: 2   Prep time: 15 minutes   Cook time: 15 minutes

This recipe will satisfy your pizza craving without all the gut-busting ingredients. The aged cheeses offer ample probiotics, and mushrooms and eggplant pack in prebiotics and nutrients.

Pinch salt

1 medium eggplant, cut into ⅛-inch slices

1 cup sliced mushrooms

1 tablespoon olive oil

1 teaspoon minced garlic

1 teaspoon Italian seasoning

1 cup shredded cheddar cheese

¼ cup shredded Parmesan cheese

1 ounce uncured all-natural pepperoni slices

1. Preheat the oven to 450°F. Line a baking sheet with parchment paper.
2. Sprinkle salt on both sides of the eggplant slices and space them out on the parchment paper. Set aside for 10 to 15 minutes.
3. Pat the eggplant dry on both sides with a paper towel. Place the mushroom slices between the eggplant slices on the baking sheet.
4. Brush the eggplant and mushrooms with olive oil and top with minced garlic.
5. Bake for 7 to 8 minutes, or until the eggplant is sizzling and lightly browned.
6. Remove the baking sheet from the oven and brush the eggplant and mushrooms with olive oil again. Sprinkle the Italian seasoning over everything.
7. Top with the cheddar, Parmesan, and pepperoni.
8. Bake again for another 3 to 4 minutes, or until the cheese is sizzling.

Per serving: Calories: 362; Fat: 26g; Protein: 18g; Carbohydrates: 16g; Fiber: 7g; Sodium: 651mg; Iron: 1mg

ROASTED VEGETABLES AND SAUSAGE

Serves: 4   **Prep time:** 10 minutes   **Cook time:** 20 minutes

This satisfying and nourishing dish comes together quickly on a busy weeknight. Fennel is great for IBS, and the garlic, vegetables, and sauerkraut support a healthy microbiome. Try to find sausages with herbs such as lemongrass and ginger to add interesting flavors and antioxidants, too.

1 small sweet potato, cubed

2 small red potatoes, cubed

1½ cups fresh green beans, cut into 2-inch pieces

1 medium onion, chopped

12 ounces all-natural sausage, cut into ½-inch slices

1 tablespoon minced garlic

2 tablespoons extra-virgin olive oil

2 teaspoons fennel seeds, crushed

½ teaspoon freshly ground black pepper

½ bunch lacinato kale, ribs removed, torn into bite-size pieces

½ cup raw sauerkraut

1. Preheat the oven to 400°F. Line two baking sheets with parchment paper.
2. Put the sweet potato, red potatoes, green beans, onion, and sausage on the prepared baking sheets, mixing and evenly dividing between the pans for even cooking.
3. In a small bowl, combine the garlic, olive oil, fennel, and pepper.
4. Add half of the oil mixture to each sheet pan and toss to coat all the sausage and vegetables.
5. Bake for 10 minutes, with each pan on different shelves in the oven.
6. Add the kale and bake for another 5 to 7 minutes, swapping the position of the sheet pans. Keep an eye on the kale so it doesn't burn. Remove from the oven and mix in the sauerkraut.

Per serving: Calories: 486; Fat: 30g; Protein: 18g; Carbohydrates: 37g; Fiber: 6g; Sodium: 752mg; Iron: 3mg

REUBEN-INSPIRED MEAT LOAF

Serves: 6   **Prep time:** 15 minutes   **Cook time:** 50 minutes

Inspired by the classic Reuben sandwich but without the inflammatory ingredients, this meat loaf goes well with a side of potatoes, sautéed spinach, or a green salad. If possible, use 100 percent grass-finished beef, which contains more gut-friendly omega-3s, antioxidants, and vitamins than standard beef. Try kimchi instead of sauerkraut if you like a little spice.

1½ pounds grass-finished ground beef

½ teaspoon salt

2 tablespoons coconut flour

1½ teaspoons fennel seeds

1 teaspoon caraway seeds

1 large egg

½ cup raw sauerkraut, finely chopped

½ sweet onion, finely chopped

½ teaspoon garlic powder

1 tablespoon Dijon mustard

1. Preheat the oven to 325°F. Line a baking sheet with foil or parchment paper.

2. In a large bowl, combine the beef, salt, coconut flour, fennel seeds, caraway seeds, egg, sauerkraut, onion, garlic powder, and mustard and mix thoroughly using your hands.

3. On the foil, shape the meat loaf into a rectangle about 1½ inches thick, 6 inches wide, and 10 inches long.

4. Bake for about 50 minutes, or until the meat is cooked through.

5. Remove the meat loaf from the oven and tent it under foil, allowing it to rest for 10 minutes.

6. Serve topped with a little extra sauerkraut, if desired.

Tip: Omit the egg if you are allergic or sensitive to them.

Per serving: Calories: 305; Fat: 23g; Protein: 20g; Carbohydrates: 3g; Fiber: 1g; Sodium: 303mg; Iron: 2mg

SHEPHERD'S PIE

Serves: 8   **Prep time:** 10 minutes   **Cook time:** 40 minutes

Containing bone broth for extra gut-healing glutamine and mushrooms and olives for extra prebiotics, this recipe is both delicious and nourishing. The cultured sour cream helps supports a healthy microbiome, too. Substituting peppers and mushrooms for the more traditional peas and carrots reduces the heavy carbohydrate load of the dish.

1½ pounds grass-finished ground beef

1 sweet onion, chopped

1 poblano chile, chopped

1 cup chopped carrots

1½ cups mushrooms, sliced

½ cup kalamata olives, sliced

1 tablespoon minced garlic

1 teaspoon dried rosemary

2 teaspoons dried oregano

1 teaspoon salt, divided

1½ tablespoons tomato paste

1 tablespoon gluten-free Worcestershire sauce

3 large russet potatoes, peeled and cut into 1-inch cubes

1¼ cups bone broth

1 heaping teaspoon cornstarch

¾ cup cultured sour cream

1. Preheat the oven to 400°F.

2. In a large ovenproof skillet over medium heat, brown the ground beef and the onion, about 8 minutes.

3. Add the poblano, carrots, mushrooms, olives, garlic, rosemary, oregano, ½ teaspoon of salt, tomato paste, and Worcestershire sauce. Cook for another 4 to 5 minutes, or until the mushrooms have softened.

4. Meanwhile, in a medium saucepan, cover the potatoes with water and bring to a boil. Reduce the heat to low and simmer for about 10 minutes, or until the potatoes are softened.

5. In a small bowl, whisk together the bone broth and cornstarch. Pour it into the meat mixture and stir.

6. Drain the potatoes, then return them to the pot and mash them with a potato masher or a fork. Mix in the sour cream and the remaining ½ teaspoon of salt.

7. Spread the potatoes over the meat mixture in an even layer. Bake for 20 to 25 minutes, or until the potatoes are lightly browned and bubbly.

Tip: Use nondairy sour cream if you are allergic or sensitive to dairy.

Per serving: Calories: 405; Fat: 23g; Protein: 20g; Carbohydrates: 31g; Fiber: 3g; Sodium: 574mg; Iron: 3mg

Measurement Conversions

	US STANDARD	US STANDARD (OUNCES)	METRIC (APPROXIMATE)
VOLUME EQUIVALENTS (LIQUID)	2 tablespoons	1 fl. oz.	30 mL
	¼ cup	2 fl. oz.	60 mL
	½ cup	4 fl. oz.	120 mL
	1 cup	8 fl. oz.	240 mL
	1½ cups	12 fl. oz.	355 mL
	2 cups or 1 pint	16 fl. oz.	475 mL
	4 cups or 1 quart	32 fl. oz.	1 L
	1 gallon	128 fl. oz.	4 L
VOLUME EQUIVALENTS (DRY)	⅛ teaspoon		0.5 mL
	¼ teaspoon		1 mL
	½ teaspoon		2 mL
	¾ teaspoon		4 mL
	1 teaspoon		5 mL
	1 tablespoon		15 mL
	¼ cup		59 mL
	⅓ cup		79 mL
	½ cup		118 mL
	⅔ cup		156 mL
	¾ cup		177 mL
	1 cup		235 mL
	2 cups or 1 pint		475 mL
	3 cups		700 mL
	4 cups or 1 quart		1 L
	½ gallon		2 L
	1 gallon		4 L
WEIGHT EQUIVALENTS	½ ounce		15 g
	1 ounce		30 g
	2 ounces		60 g
	4 ounces		115 g
	8 ounces		225 g
	12 ounces		340 g
	16 ounces or 1 pound		455 g

	FAHRENHEIT (F)	CELSIUS (C) (APPROXIMATE)
OVEN TEMPERATURES	250°F	120°C
	300°F	150°C
	325°F	180°C
	375°F	190°C
	400°F	200°C
	425°F	220°C
	450°F	230°C

Resources

Dr. Mark Hyman: Dr. Mark Hyman is an internationally recognized expert in functional medicine. He has books, recipes, and a podcast called *The Doctor's Farmacy*. DrHyman.com/about

***The Healthy RD* (blog)**: The Healthy RD is my website. It has in-depth blog posts about a variety of gut health topics, such as the auto-immune protocol diet, how ox bile works, the mitochondria diet, medicinal mushrooms, and more. TheHealthyRD.com

***Brain Maker: The Power of Gut Microbes to Heal and Protect Your Brain–for Life* by David Perlmutter, MD**: *Brain Maker* is a book written by Dr. David Perlmutter, a board-certified neurologist and published researcher and author.

Montana Functional Health: Dr. Heather Maddox, Lindsay Peterson, FNP, and their team offer great blog articles about gut health. MFHCare.com

The National Library of Medicine: Contains research papers about gut health and many other health tips. NCBI.NLM.NIH.gov

***The Wahls Protocol: A Radical New Way to Treat All Chronic Auto-immune Conditions Using Paleo Principles* by Terry Wahls, MD**: Dr. Wahls became an expert in gut health after she developed debilitating multiple sclerosis and found that food has been the biggest factor in healing. TerryWahls.com

References

Acalovschi, Monica, and Frank Lammert. "The Growing Global Burden of Gallstone Disease." (2020) *World Journal of Gastroenterology*. WorldGastroenterology.org/publications/e-wgn/e-wgn-expert-point -of-view-articles-collection/the-growing-global-burden-of-gallstone -disease.

Akbari, Elmira, Zatollah Asemi, Reza Daneshvar Kakhaki, Fereshteh Bahmani, Ebrahim Kouchaki, Omid Reza Tamtaji, Gholam Ali Hamidi, and Mahmoud Salami. (November 2016) "Effect of Probi- otic Supplementation on Cognitive Function and Metabolic Status in Alzheimer's Disease: A Randomized, Double-Blind and Con- trolled Trial." *Frontiers in Aging Neuroscience* 8 (256). DOI: 10.3389 /fnagi.2016.00256.

Akram, Farooq, Yufang Huang, Valencia Lim, Paul J. Huggan, and Reshma A. Merchant. (November 2014) "Proton Pump Inhibitors: Are We Still Prescribing Them Without Valid Indications?" *Australasian Medical Journal* 7 (11): 465–470. DOI: 10.4066 /AMJ.2014.2093.

Al-Howiriny, Tawfeq, Abdulmalik Alsheikh, Saleh Alqasoumi, Mohammed Al-Yahya, Kamal El–Tahir, and Syed Rafatullah. (July 2010) "Gastric Antiulcer, Antisecretory and Cytoprotective Proper- ties of Celery (Apium Graveolens) in Rats." *Pharmaceutical Biology* 48 (7): 786–793. DOI: 10.3109/13880200903280026.

American Institute of Stress. "Stress Research." (2020). Stress.org /stress-research.

Balfegó, Mariona, Silvia Canivell, Felicia A. Hanzu, Aleix Sala-Vila, Margarita Martínez-Medina, Serafín Murillo, Teresa Mur, et al. (April 2016) "Effects of Sardine-Enriched Diet on Metabolic Control, Inflammation and Gut Microbiota in Drug-Naïve Patients with Type 2 Diabetes: A Pilot Randomized Trial." *Lipids in Health and Disease* 15 (78). DOI: 10.1186/s12944-016-0245-0.

Bischoff, Stephan C., Giovanni Barbara, Wim Buurman, Theo Ockhuizen, Jörg-Dieter Schulzke, Matteo Serino, Herbert Tilg, et al. "Intestinal Permeability: A New Target for Disease Prevention and Therapy." *BMC Gastroenterology* 14, no. 189 (November 2014). DOI: 10.1186/s12876-014-0189-7.

Bisht, Babita, Warren G. Darling, Ruth E. Grossmann, E. Torage Shivapour, Susan K. Lutgendorf, Linda G. Snetselaar, Michael J. Hall, et al. (May 2014) "A Multimodal Intervention for Patients with Secondary Progressive Multiple Sclerosis: Feasibility and Effect on Fatigue." *Journal of Alternative and Complementary Medicine* 20 (5): 347–355. DOI: 10.1089/acm.2013.0188.

Bressa, Carlo, María Bailén-Andrino, Jennifer Pérez-Santiago, Rocío González-Soltero, Margarita Pérez, Maria Gregoria Montalvo-Lominchar, Jose Luis Maté-Muñoz, et al. (February 2017) "Differences in Gut Microbiota Profile Between Women with Active Lifestyle and Sedentary Women." *PLoS One* 12 (2): e0171352. DOI: 10.1371/journal.pone.0171352.

Camara-Lemarroy, Carlos R., Luanne M. Metz, and V. Wee Yong. (October 2018) "Focus on the Gut-Brain Axis: Multiple Sclerosis, the Intestinal Barrier and the Microbiome." *World Journal of Gastroenterology* 24 (37): 4271–4223. DOI: 10.3748/wjg.v24.i37.4217.

Chandrasekaran, Anita, Shauna Groven, James D. Lewis, Susan S. Levy, Caroline Diamant, Emily Singh, and Gauree Gupta Konijeti. (October 2019) "An Autoimmune Protocol Diet Improves Patient-Reported Quality of Life in Inflammatory Bowel Disease." *Crohns & Colitis 360* 1 (3). DOI: 10.1093/crocol/otz01.

Chassaing, Benoit, Tom Van de Wiele, Jana De Bodt, Massimo Marzorati, and Andrew T. Gewirtz. (August 2017) "Dietary Emulsifiers Directly Alter Human Microbiota Composition and Gene Expression *Ex Vivo* Potentiating Intestinal Inflammation." *Gut* 66 (8): 1414–1427. DOI: 10.1136/gutjnl-2016-313099.

Chen, Jingyuan, Yuan Guo, Yajun Gui, and Danyan Xu. (January 2018) "Physical Exercise, Gut, Gut Microbiota, and Atherosclerotic Cardiovascular Diseases." *Lipids in Health and Disease* 17 (1). DOI: 10.1186/s12944-017-0653-9.

Chonpathompikunlert, Pennapa, Phetcharat Boonruamkaew, Wanida Sukketsiri, Pilaiwanwadee Hutamekalin, and Morakot Sroyraya. (March 2018) "The Antioxidant and Neurochemical Activity of *Apium Graveolens* L. and its Ameliorative Effect on MPTP-Induced Parkinson-Like Symptoms in Mice." *BMC Complementary and Alternative Medicine* 18 (1): 103. DOI: 10.1186/s12906-018-2166-0.

Clapp, Megan, Nadia Aurora, Lindsey Herrera, Manisha Bhatia, Emily Wilen, and Sarah Wakefield. (September 2017) "Gut Microbiota's Effect on Mental Health: The Gut-Brain Axis." *The International Journal of Clinical Practice* 7 (4): 987. DOI: 10.4081/cp.2017.987.

Cui, Bo, Donghong Su, Wenlong Li, Xiaojun She, Ming Zhang, Rui Wang, and Qingfeng Zhai. (June 2018) "Effects of Chronic Noise Exposure on the Microbiome-Gut-Brain Axis in Senescence-Accelerated Prone Mice: Implications for Alzheimer's Disease." *Journal of Neuroinflammation* 15 (1): 190. DOI: 10.1186/s12974-018-1223-4.

Den, Haoyue, Xunhu Dong, Mingliang Chen, and Zhongmin Zou. (February 2020) "Efficacy of Probiotics on Cognition, and Biomarkers of Inflammation and Oxidative Stress in Adults with Alzheimer's Disease or Mild Cognitive Impairment: A Meta-Analysis of Randomized Controlled Trials." *Aging* 12 (4): 4010–4039. DOI: 10.18632/aging.102810.

Fasano, Alessio. (January 2020) "All Disease Begins in the (Leaky) Gut: Role of Zonulin Mediated Gut Permeability in the Pathogenesis of Some Chronic Inflammatory Diseases." *F1000Research* 9. DOI: 10.12688/f1000research.20510.1.

Ghevariya, Vishal, Shashideep Singhal, and Sury Anand. (July 2013) "The Skin: A Mirror to the Gut." *International Journal of Colorectal Disease* 28 (7): 889–913. DOI: 10.1007/s00384-012-1637-x.

Gilani, Anwarul Hassan, Qaiser Jabeen, Arif-ullah Khan, and Abdul Jabbar Shah. (February 2007) "Gut Modulatory, Blood Pressure Lowering, Diuretic and Sedative Activities of Cardamom." *Journal of Ethnopharmacology* 115 (3): 463–472. DOI: 10.1016/j.jep .2007.10.015.

Giloteaux, Ludovic, Julia K. Goodrich, William A. Walters, Susan M. Levine, Ruth E. Ley, and Maureen R. Hanson. (2016) "Reduced Diversity and Altered Composition of the Gut Microbiome in Individuals with Myalgic Encephalomyelitis/Chronic Fatigue Syndrome." *Microbiome* 4 (30). DOI: 10.1186/s40168-016-0171-4.

Hevia, Arancha, Susana Delgado, Borja Sánchez, and Abelardo Margolles. (November 2015) "Molecular Players Involved in the Interaction Between Beneficial Bacteria and the Immune System." *Frontiers in Microbiology* 6: 1285. DOI: 10.3389/fmicb.2015.01285.

Houghton, Christine A. (2019) "Sulforaphane: Its 'Coming of Age' as a Clinically Relevant Nutraceutical in the Prevention and Treatment of Chronic Disease." *Oxidative Medicine and Cellular Longevity* (2019): 2716870. DOI: 10.1155/2019/2716870.

Ianiro, Gianluca, Silvia Pecere, Valentina Giorgio, Antonio Gasbarrini, and Giovanni Cammarota. (February 2016) "Digestive Enzyme Supplementation in Gastrointestinal Diseases." *Current Drug Metabolism* 17 (2): 187–193. DOI: 10.2174/138920021702160 114150137.

Ina, Kenji, Ryuichi Furuta, Takae Kataoka, Satoshi Kayukawa, Takashi Yoshida, Takaya Miwa, Yoshitaka Yamamura, et al. (October 2011) "Lentinan Prolonged Survival in Patients with Gastric Cancer Receiving S-1-Based Chemotherapy." *World Journal of Clinical Oncology* 2 (10): 339–343. DOI: 10.5306/wjco.v2.i10.339.

Jamal, A., K. Javed, M. Aslam, and M. A. Jafri. (January 2006) "Gas-troprotective Effect of Cardamom, *Elettaria Cardamomum* Maton. Fruits in Rats." *Journal of Ethnopharmacology* 103 (2): 149–153. DOI: 10.1016/j.jep.2005.07.016.

Jiao, Yuhao, Li Wu, Nicholas D. Huntington N, and Xuan Zhang. (February 2020) "Crosstalk Between Gut Microbiota and Innate Immunity and Its Implication in Autoimmune Diseases." *Frontiers in Immunology* 11: 282. DOI: 10.3389/fimmu.2020.00282.

Kanai, Takanori, Katsuyoshi Matsuoka, Makoto Naganuma, Atsushi Hayashi, and Tadakazu Hisamatsu. (July 2014) "Diet, Microbiota, and Inflammatory Bowel Disease: Lessons from Japanese Foods." *The Korean Journal of Internal Medicine* 29 (4): 409–415. DOI: 10.3904/kjim.2014.29.4.409.

Konijeti, Gauree G., NaMee Kim, James D. Lewis, Shauna Groven, Anita Chandrasekaran, Sirisha Grandhe, Caroline Diamant, et al. (November 2017) "Efficacy of the Autoimmune Protocol Diet for Inflammatory Bowel Disease." *Inflammatory Bowel Disease* 23 (11): 2054–2060. DOI: 10.1097/MIB.0000000000001221.

Kuttner, Leora, Christine T. Chambers, Janine Hardial, David M. Israel, Kevan Jacobson, and Kathy Evans. (2006) "A Randomized Trial of Yoga for Adolescents with Irritable Bowel Syndrome." *Pain Research and Management* 11 (4): 217–223. DOI: 10.1155/2006/731628.

Markowiak, Paulina, and Katarzyna Śliżewska. (September 2017) "Effects of Probiotics, Prebiotics, and Synbiotics on Human Health." *Nutrients* 9 (9): 1021. DOI: 10.3390/nu9091021.

Morshedi, Mohammad, Reza Hashemi, Sara Moazzen, Amirhossein Sahebkar, and Elaheh-Sadat Hosseinifard. (November 2019) "Immunomodulatory and Anti-Inflammatory Effects of Probiotics in Multiple Sclerosis: A Systematic Review." *Journal of Neuroinflammation* 16 (1). DOI: 10.1186/s12974-019-1611-4.

National Institute of Mental Health. (February 2019) "Statistics: Major Depression." NIMH.NIH.gov/health/statistics/major-depression .shtml.

Ohsawa, Kazuhito, Fumiya Nakamura, Naoto Uchida, Seiichi Mizuno, and Hidehiko Yokogoshi. (May 2018) "Lactobacillus Helveticus-Fermented Milk Containing Lactononadecapeptide (NIPPLTQTPVVVPPFLQPE) Improves Cognitive Function in Healthy Middle-Aged Adults: A Randomised, Double-Blind, Placebo-Controlled Trial." *International Journal of Food Sciences and Nutrition* 69 (3): 369–376. DOI: 10.1080 /09637486.2017.1365824.

Prakash, U. N., and K. Srinivasan. (July 2013) "Enhanced Intestinal Uptake of Iron, Zinc and Calcium in Rats Fed Pungent Spice Principles—Piperine, Capsaicin and Ginger (Zingiber Offici- nale)." *Journal of Trace Elements in Medicine and Biology* 27 (3): 184–190. DOI: 10.1016/j.jtemb.2012.11.003.

Qi, Dan, Xiao-Lu Nie, and Jian-Jun Zhang. (April 2020) "The Effect of Probiotics Supplementation on Blood Pressure: A Systemic Review and Meta-Analysis." *Lipids in Health and Disease* 19 (1): 79. DOI: 10.1186/s12944-020-01259-x.

Quave, Cassandra. (2020) "Expert Q&A: Explore Why the Skin's Delicate Ecosystem Depends on a Healthy Microbiome." *Medline.* Medline.com/skin-health/skin-microbiome.

Raygan, Fariba, Zohreh Rezavandi, Fereshteh Bahmani, Vahi- dreza Ostadmohammadi, Mohammad Ali Mansournia, Maryam Tajabadi-Ebrahimi, Shokoofeh Borzabadi, et al. (June 2018) "The Effects of Probiotic Supplementation on Metabolic Status in Type 2 Diabetic Patients with Coronary Heart Disease." *Diabetology and Metabolic Syndrome* 10 (51). DOI: 10.1186/s13098-018-0353-2.

Ruixue Huang, Ruixue, Ke Wang, and Jianan Hu. (August 2016) "Effect of Probiotics on Depression: A Systematic Review and

Meta-Analysis of Randomized Controlled Trials." *Nutrients* 8 (8): 483. DOI: 10.3390/nu8080483.

Saulnier, Delphine M., Yehuda Ringel, Melvin B. Heyman, Jane A. Foster, Premysl Bercik, Robert J. Shulman, James Versalovic, et al. (January 2013) "The Intestinal Microbiome, Probiotics and Prebiotics in Neurogastroenterology." *Gut Microbes* 4 (1): 17–27. DOI: 10.4161/gmic.22973.

Scott, Alasdair J., Claire A. Merrifield, Jessica A. Younes, and Elizabeth P. Pekelharing. (September 2018) "Pre-, Pro- and Synbiotics in Cancer Prevention and Treatment—A Review of Basic and Clinical Research." *Ecancermedicalscience* 12: 869. DOI: 10.3332/ecancer.2018.869.

Smith, Robert P., Cole Easson, Sarah M. Lyle, Ritishka Kapoor, Chase P. Donnelly, Eileen J. Davidson, Esha Parikh, et al. (October 2019) "Gut Microbiome Diversity is Associated with Sleep Physiology in Humans." *PLoS One* 14 (10): e0222394. DOI: 10.1371/journal.pone.0222394.

Tang, Yao, Juan Huang, Wen Yue Zhang, Si Qin, Yi Xuan Yang, Hong Ren, Qin-bing Yang, et al. (September 2019) "Effects of Probiotics on Nonalcoholic Fatty Liver Disease: A Systematic Review and Meta-Analysis." *Therapeutic Advances in Gastroenterology* 12 (3): 1756284819878046. DOI: 10.1177/1756284819878046.

Touret, Tiago, Manuela Oliveira, and Teresa Semedo-Lemsaddek. (September 2018) "Putative Probiotic Lactic Acid Bacteria Isolated from Sauerkraut Fermentations." *PLoS One* 13 (9): e0203501. DOI: 10.1371/journal.pone.0203501.

Tuck, Caroline J., Jessica R. Biesiekierski, Peter Schmid-Grendelmeier, and Daniel Pohl. (July 2019) "Food Intolerances." *Nutrients* 11 (7): 1684. DOI: 10.3390/nu11071684.

Turati, Federica, Claudio Pelucchi, Valentina Guercio, Carlo La Vecchia, and Carlotta Galeone. (January 2015) "Allium Vegetable Intake and Gastric Cancer: A Case-Control Study and Meta-Analysis." *Molecular Nutrition & Food Research* 59 (1): 171–179. DOI: 10.1002/mnfr.201400496.

Vamanua, Emanuel, and Diana Pelinescu. (November 2017) "Effects of Mushroom Consumption on the Microbiota of Different Target Groups–Impact of Polyphenolic Composition and Mitigation on the Microbiome Fingerprint." *LWT–Food Science and Technology* Part A, 85: 262–268. DOI: 10.1016/j.lwt.2017.07.039.

Vitetta, Luis, Gemma Vitetta, and Sean Hall. (October 2018) "Immunological Tolerance and Function: Associations Between Intestinal Bacteria, Probiotics, Prebiotics, and Phages." *Frontiers in Immunology* 9: 2240. DOI: 10.3389/fimmu.2018.02240.

Walter, S. A., M. P. Jones, N. J. Talley, L. Kjellström, H. Nyhlin, A. N. Andreasson, and L. Agréus. (September 2013) "Abdominal Pain is Associated with Anxiety and Depression Scores in a Sample of the General Adult Population with No Signs of Organic Gastrointestinal Disease." *Journal of Neurogastroenterology and Motility* 25 (9): 741–e576. DOI: 10.1111/nmo.12155.

Wang, Hui, Yong Cai, Yue Zheng, Qixuan Bai, Dongling Xie, and Jiufei Yu. (October 2017) "Efficacy of Biological Response Modifier Lentinan with Chemotherapy for Advanced Cancer: A Meta-Analysis." *Cancer Medicine* 6 (10): 2222–2233. DOI: 10.1002/cam4.1156.

World Health Organization. (February 2018) "Physical Activity." WHO.int/news-room/fact-sheets/detail/physical-activity.

Yanaka, Akinori. (January 2018) "Daily Intake of Broccoli Sprouts Normalizes Bowel Habits in Human Healthy Subjects." *Journal of Clinical Biochemistry and Nutrition* 62 (1): 75–82. DOI: 10.3164/jcbn.17-42.

Yang, Beibei, Jinbao Wei, Peijun Ju, and Jinghong Chen. (May 2019) "Effects of Regulating Intestinal Microbiota on Anxiety Symptoms: A Systematic Review. *General Psychiatry* 32 (2). DOI: 10.1136 /gpsych-2019-100056.

Index

R

Rebalance principle, 8, 40
Remove principle, 8
Repair principle, 8
Replace principle, 8
Repopulate principle, 8
Reuben-Inspired Meat Loaf, 141
Revolved chair twist, 45–46
Rice, Fried, with Vegetables,
    Fermented, 136–137
Roasted Almond and Maple-
    Broccoli Salad, 108–109
Roasted Vegetables and Sausage, 140

S

Salads
    Basil, Tomato, and Cucumber
        Quinoa Salad, 110–111
    Beet and Mint Salad, 96
    Crunchy Curry Celery Salad, 101
    Fresh Greens and Salmon Salad, 98–99
    Lemon, Parmesan, and Kale Salad, 107
    Roasted Almond and Maple-
        Broccoli Salad, 108–109
    Sauerkraut and Bell Pepper Salad, 100
    Yogurt Berry Salad, 102
Saliva, 2
Salmon
    Fresh Greens and Salmon Salad, 98–99
    Mediterranean Salmon, 120
    Salmon and Fennel Scramble, 90
    Salmon Burrito Bowls, 121
Salmon and Fennel Scramble, 90
Sardines, 34
Sauerkraut, 33
    Cod with Sauerkraut, 123
    Reuben-Inspired Meat Loaf, 141
    Sauerkraut and Bell Pepper Salad, 100
Sausage
    Breakfast Bake, 92
    Roasted Vegetables and Sausage, 140
Sautéed Brussels Sprouts and Herbs, 112
Sealey, Michael, 48

Shepherd's Pie, 142–143
Shrimp
    Ginger Shrimp Stir-Fry, 122
    Shrimp Enchiladas, 124–125
Sides
    Curry Cauliflower Pickles, 106
    Pickled Carrots and Onions, 97
    Sautéed Brussels Sprouts
        and Herbs, 112
    Stuffed Mushrooms, 105
    Sweet Potato Fries, 104
Skin health, 7, 14
Sleep, 47
Smoothies
    Chocolate-Spinach Smoothie, 80
    Lemon-Ginger Smoothie, 79
    Vibrant Green Smoothie, 78
Soups
    Carrot, Ginger, and Fennel Soup, 113
    Chicken Noodle Soup, 115
    Ginger and Coriander Vegetable
        Beef Soup, 116
    Hot and Sour Mushroom
        Vegetable Soup, 114
Spiced Turkey Meatballs, 138
Spices, 24
Spinach
    Chocolate-Spinach Smoothie, 80
    Vibrant Green Smoothie, 78
Stew, Beef and Vegetable, 134
Stir-Fry, Ginger Shrimp, 122
Stomach, 2
Strength-building exercises, 42
Stress, 52–53
Stress hormones, 41, 52
Stress management, 54–55
Stuffed Mushrooms, 105
Substitutions, 35, 65
Sunflower-Ginger Cereal, 83
Sunlight, 47
Sunrise Lemon-Chia Pudding, 81
Supine twist, 45
Supplements, 25, 35–36, 70

Acknowledgments

Writing has always been a passion of mine, so pursuing this book has brought me a lot of joy. For this reason, I want to thank the publisher and the editor of this book for allowing me to share compelling research about gut health with you. From the time I was small, I enjoyed putting pencil to paper (now clicking the keys) as my thoughts poured out.

I want to thank my many friends for encouraging me along the way. From beginning to end, they cheered me on. No matter what adventures I take on, they have my back.

Even though they are quite a distance away, my parents are always supportive of me. They even taste-tested and inspired some of the recipes. They have always been my rock.

Finally, my husband, Tony Moretti, and two kids, Dante and Josie, who were very supportive of me and always (somewhat!) willing to try my new recipes. I sometimes kept them awake with typing while working on this book and it even interrupted our evening relaxation time, so I thank them for being patient.

About the Author

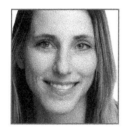

Heidi Moretti, MS, RD, is a writer and blogger with the website *The Healthy RD* and cowriter of *Thyroid Nutrition Educators*. She has been a practicing clinical registered dietitian for 21 years, much of that with Providence St. Patrick Hospital and most recently with Fresenius Kidney Care. Heidi has a passion for putting more healing into medicine by using functional nutrition, holistic health, and natural medicine to get to the root causes of illnesses.

Heidi received a master of science in nutritional science from the University of Washington. A registered and licensed dietitian, Heidi has a passion for improving vitality through food. When Heidi was pursuing her undergraduate studies at Montana State University, one of her professors, Melody Anacker, MS, RDN, made her begin to understand that healing begins with the food we eat.

Heidi has researched vitamins, supplements, and food as medicine throughout her career, and her research has been published in peer-reviewed journals like *Journal of Renal Nutrition* and *BMC Cardiovascular Disorders*.

CPSIA information can be obtained
at www.ICGtesting.com
Printed in the USA
BVHW021438250122
626961BV00001BA/1